ORTHOPEDIC CLINICS OF NORTH AMERICA

www.orthopedic.theclinics.com

Regenerative Medicine

October 2026 • Volume 57 • Number 4

ELSEVIER

1818 Market Street • Suite 3323 • Philadelphia, Pennsylvania, 19103-2899.

http://www.orthopedic.theclinics.com

ORTHOPEDIC CLINICS OF NORTH AMERICA Volume 57, Number 4
October 2026 ISSN 0030-5898, ISBN-13: 978-0-443-43098-5

Editor: Megan Ashdown
Developmental Editor: Sukirti Singh

Publishing Office: *Orthopedic Clinics of North America* (ISSN 0030-5898) is published quarterly by Elsevier Inc., 1818 Market Street, Philadelphia, PA 19103, United States. Periodicals postage paid at New York, NY and additional mailing offices. USA POSTMASTER: Send address changes to *Orthopedic Clinics of North America*, Elsevier Customer Service Department, 3251 Riverport Lane, Maryland Heights, MO 63043, USA. Months of issue are January, April, July, and October. Subscription prices are $376.00 per year for (US individuals), $437.00 per year (Canadian individuals), $516.00 per year (international individuals), $100.00 per year (US students), $100.00 per year for (Canadian students), $220.00 per year for (international students). For institutional access pricing please contact Customer Service via the contact information below. Foreign air speed delivery is included in all *Clinics* subscription prices. All prices are subject to change without notice. Orders, claims, and journal inquiries: Please visit our Support Hub page https://service.elsevier.com for assistance.

Reprints. For copies of 100 or more, of articles in this publication, please contact the Commercial Reprints Department, Elsevier Inc., 360 Park Avenue South, New York, NY 10010-1710. Tel.: 212-633-3874; Fax: 212-633-3820; E-mail: reprints@elsevier.com.

Orthopedic Clinics of North America is covered in *MEDLINE/PubMed* (*Index Medicus*), *Cinahl, Excerpta Medica, and Cumulative Index to Nursing and Allied Health Literature.*

EDITORIAL BOARD

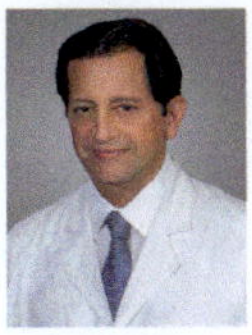

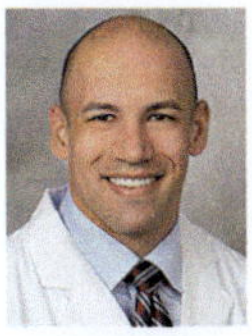

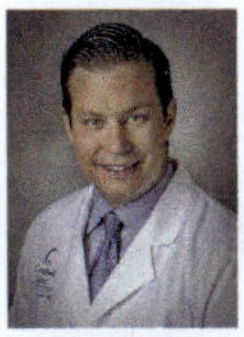

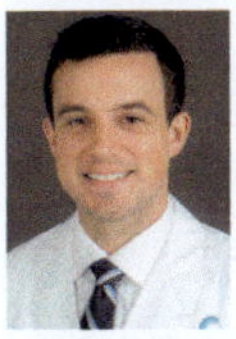

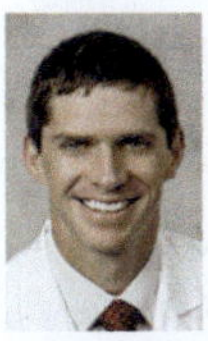

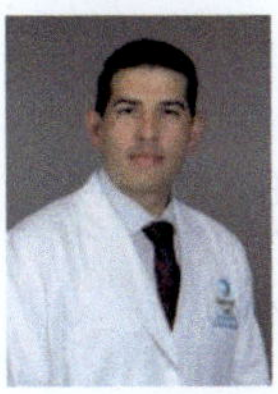

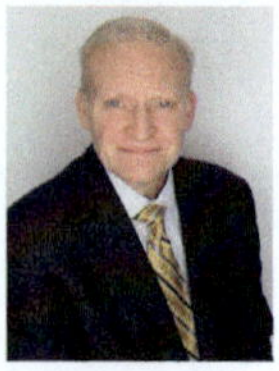

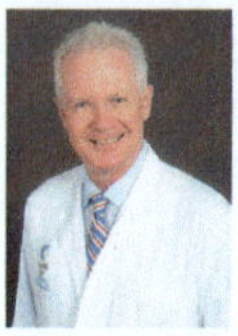

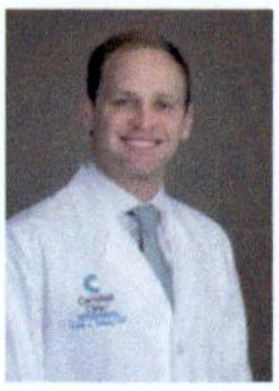

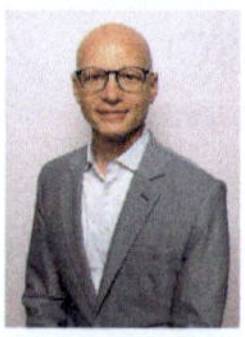

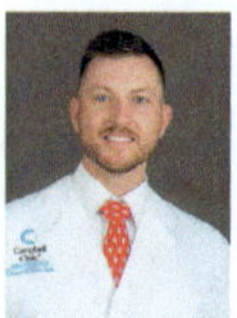

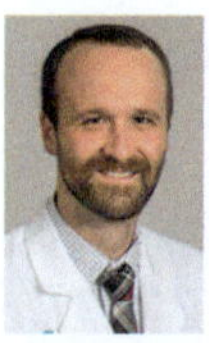

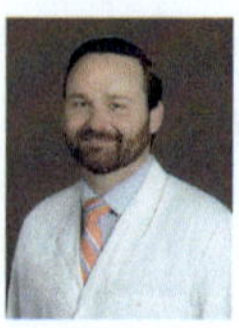

CONTRIBUTORS

EDITOR

FREDERICK M. AZAR, MD
Harold B. Boyd Professor and Chair, Director, Sports Medicine Fellowship, University of Tennessee Health Science Center – Campbell Clinic, Department of Orthopaedic Surgery and Biomedical Engineering, Memphis, Tennessee, USA

AUTHORS

JESSALYNN ADAM, MD, FAAPMR, CAQSM
Clinical Instructor, Department of Family Medicine, National Capital Sports Medicine Consortium, Bethesda, Maryland, USA; Private Practice, Sports Medicine Physiatrist, OrthoVirginia, Alexandria, Virginia, USA; Head Team Physician, DC Power, Washington, DC, USA

SUNEEL S. APTE, MBBS, DPhil
Research Scientist, Department of Biomedical Engineering, Lerner Research Institute, Cleveland Clinic, Cleveland, Ohio, USA

ALYSSA BARRÉ, MD
Resident Physician, PGY-4, Department of Orthopaedic Surgery and Sports Medicine, University of Kentucky, Lexington, Kentucky, USA

TAEWOONG CHAE, MD
Resident, Department of Orthopaedics, University of British Columbia, Vancouver, Canada

CHRISTOPHER COSGROVE, MD
Assistant Professor, Department of Orthopaedic Surgery & Biomedical Engineering, The University of Tennessee Health Science Center (UTHSC) - Campbell Clinic; Staff Physician, Campbell Clinic, Inc, Memphis, Tennessee, USA

KATHLEEN DERWIN, PhD
Research Scientist, Department of Biomedical Engineering, Lerner Research Institute, Vice Chair, Innovation Management and Conflict of Interest, Co-Director, Musculoskeletal Research Center, Cleveland Clinic, Cleveland, Ohio, USA

GARRY W.K. HO, MD, FACSM, FAMSSM, FAAFP, CAQSM, RMSK
Associate Professor of Medical Education, Office of Educational Affairs, University of Virginia School of Medicine, Charlottesville, Virginia, USA; Adjunct Associate Clinical Professor, Department of Family Medicine, Uniformed Services University of the Health Sciences, Bethesda, Maryland, USA; Associate Clinical Professor, Department of Family Medicine, Clinical Teaching Faculty, University of Virginia School of Medicine, Northern Virginia Division, Inova Campus, Fairfax, Virginia, USA; Adjunct Associate Clinical Professor, Department of Family Medicine, Virginia Commonwealth University School of Medicine, Richmond, Virginia, USA; Adjunct Associate Clinical Professor, Department of Family Medicine, Georgetown University School of Medicine, Washington, DC, USA; Team Physician, George Mason University, Fairfax, Virginia, USA; Core Faculty, MSKUS - Musculoskeletal Ultrasound, Visa, California, USA; Clinical Instructor, National Capital Sports Medicine Consortium, Bethesda, Maryland, USA; Private Practice, Sports Medicine Physician, Interventional Sonologist, OrthoVirginia, Fairfax, Virginia, USA

CHRISTOPHER HOLLAND, MD, MS
Clinical Instructor, Department of Orthopaedic Surgery & Biomedical Engineering, The University of Tennessee Health Science Center (UTHSC) - Campbell

Clinic; Staff Physician, Campbell Clinic, Inc, Memphis, Tennessee, USA

LISA C. HOWARD, MD, MHSc, FRCSC
Assistant Professor, Department of Orthopaedics, University of British Columbia, Vancouver, Canada

DYLAN KLUCK, MD
Assistant Professor of Pediatric Orthopaedic Surgery, Department of Orthopaedic Surgery and Sports Medicine, University of Kentucky, Shriners Children's Lexington, Lexington, Kentucky, USA

XIAOJUAN LI, PhD
Research Scientist, Department of Biomedical Engineering, Lerner Research Institute, Director, Program for Advanced Musculoskeletal Imaging, Cleveland Clinic, Cleveland, Ohio, USA

BASSAM A. MASRI, MD, FRCSC
Professor, Department of Orthopaedics, University of British Columbia, Vancouver, Canada

MAX MICHALSKI, MD, MS, FAAOS
Assistant Professor, Department of Orthopaedic Surgery, Cedars Sinai Orthopaedic Center, Los Angeles, California, USA

WILLIAM M. MIHALKO, MD, PhD
Professor & J.R. Hyde Chair of Excellence, Chair Joint Graduate Program in Biomedical Engineering, Department of Orthopaedic Surgery & Biomedical Engineering, The University of Tennessee Health Science Center (UTHSC) - Campbell Clinic, Memphis, Tennessee, USA

CHARLES MOON, MD, FAAOS
Professor, Vice Chair, Director Orthopedic Trauma Orthopaedic Surgery, Department of Orthopaedic Surgery, Cedars Sinai Orthopaedic Center, Los Angeles, California, USA

MICHAEL E. NEUFELD, MD, FRCSC, MSc
Clinical Assistant Professor, Department of Orthopaedics, University of British Columbia, Vancouver, Canada

SHLOK V. PATEL, MD
Clinical Research Fellow, Department of Orthopaedic Surgery, Cleveland Clinic, Cleveland, Ohio, USA

NICOLAS S. PIUZZI, MD
Associate Professor, Department of Orthopaedic Surgery, Co-Director, Department of Biomedical Engineering, Lerner Research Institute, Cleveland Clinic, Cleveland, Ohio, USA

KRISTINA QUIROLGICO, MD, FAAPMR, CAQSM
Assistant Professor, Department of Orthopaedic Surgery and Biomedical Engineering, University of Tennessee Health Science Center, Memphis, Tennessee, USA; Sports Medicine Physiatrist, Campbell Clinic, Germantown, Tennessee, USA; Company Physician, Ballet Memphis, Memphis, Tennessee, USA

SAMUEL RASZKA, MD
Resident, Department of Orthopaedic Surgery, Cedars Sinai Orthopaedic Center, Los Angeles, California, USA

J. MICHAEL RUTH Jr, MD
Resident Physician, Department of Orthopaedic Surgery and Biomedical Engineering, Resident, University of Tennessee Health Science Center-Campbell Clinic, Memphis, Tennessee, USA

EMILY SALLADE, BS, CCRC
Clinical Research Coordinator, Acera Surgical, Inc, St Louis, Missouri, USA

OLIVIA SCHAFFER, BS
Student, Department of Orthopedic Surgery, NYU Langone, New York, New York, USA

RAN SCHWARZKOPF, MD, MSc
Professor, Department of Orthopedic Surgery, System Director of Strategic Initiatives and Operations, Julia Flesher Koch, NYU Langone, New York, New York, USA

MAXWELL TRUDEAU, MD
Resident, Department of Orthopedic Surgery, NYU Langone, New York, New York, USA

WARRAN WIGNADASAN, MBBS, BSc(Hons), FRCS(Orth)
Fellow, Department of Orthopaedics, University of British Columbia, Vancouver, Canada

CONTENTS

REGENERATIVE MEDICINE

FORTHCOMING ISSUES

January 2027
Minimally Invasive Surgery
Colin T. Ackerman, Michael J. Beebe, Christopher T. Cosgrove, Benjamin J. Grear, Austin T. Hardaway, Christopher Thomas Holland, William M. Mihalko, G. Andrew Murphy, Keith J. Orland, David R. Richardson, Carson M. Rider, and Benjamin Sheffer, *Editors*

April 2027
Complications in Orthopedic Surgery
Colin T. Ackerman, Michael J. Beebe, Christopher T. Cosgrove, Benjamin J. Grear, Austin T. Hardaway, Christopher Thomas Holland, William M. Mihalko, G. Andrew Murphy, Keith J. Orland, David R. Richardson, Carson M. Rider, and Benjamin Sheffer, *Editors*

July 2027
Imaging in Orthopedic Practice
Colin T. Ackerman, Michael J. Beebe, Christopher T. Cosgrove, Benjamin J. Grear, Austin T. Hardaway, Christopher Thomas Holland, William M. Mihalko, G. Andrew Murphy, Keith J. Orland, David R. Richardson, Carson M. Rider, and Benjamin Sheffer, *Editors*

RECENT ISSUES

July 2026
New Technologies
Frederick M. Azar, Michael J. Beebe, Tyler J. Brolin, Christopher T. Cosgrove, Benjamin J. Grear, William M. Mihalko, Benjamin Sheffer, William J. Weller, David R Richardson, Carson M. Rider, and Garnett Andrew Murphy, *Editors*

April 2026
Unique or Select Procedures
Michael J. Beebe, Tyler J. Brolin, Christopher T. Cosgrove, Benjamin J. Grear, Christopher Thomas Holland, William M. Mihalko, G. Andrew Murphy, Keith J. Orland, David R. Richardson, Carson M. Rider, Benjamin Sheffer, and William J. Weller, *Editors*

January 2026
Evidence-Based Medicine
Michael J. Beebe, Tyler J. Brolin, Christopher T. Cosgrove, Benjamin J. Grear, Christopher Thomas Holland, William M. Mihalko, Keith J. Orland, Benjamin Sheffer, Omar X. Medina, and William J. Weller, *Editors*

PREFACE

Regenerative Medicine

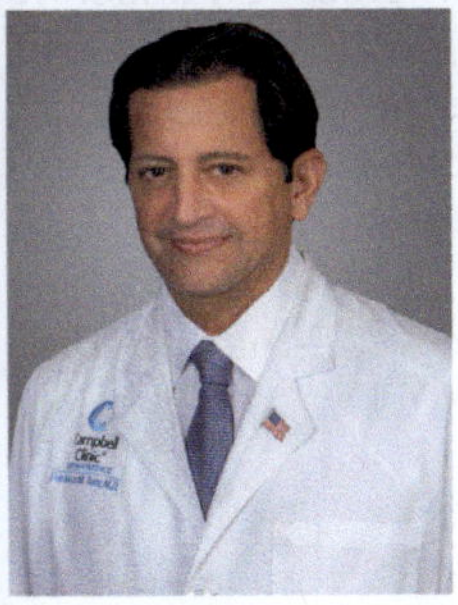

Frederick M. Azar, MD
Editor

Development of new technologies has improved the quality and delivery of patient care. This quarter, *Orthopedic Clinics of North America* focuses on regenerative medicine and the implications for orthopedic patients and surgeons.

Osteoarthritis is a common joint disorder that is influenced by many factors. In the knee and hip section, Patel and colleagues provide a thorough two-part review of osteoarthritis as a whole-joint disease. The first part of their review examines current management and the structural and mechanism-informed strategies of treatment directed at cartilage metabolism, synovitis and inflammation, and subchondral bone remodeling. In the second part, they explore therapeutic strategies that include pain pathways, systemic metabolic dysfunction, cellular aging, and contemporary regenerative therapies, such as platelet-rich plasma (PRP), hyaluronic acid, and cell-based products.

Wignadasan and colleagues continue the discussion of osteoarthritis of the knee with a review of treatment using PRP. Although generally considered safe, PRP is a costly treatment that has not yet shown consistent superior results, but it is considered an adjunct for selected patients desiring to delay surgery. Ruth and colleagues discuss advances in gene therapy and its potential to treat the underlying disease mechanisms rather than merely alleviating symptoms. And with the growth of the use of GLP-1 receptor agonist treatments for obesity, Schaffer and colleagues discuss possible musculoskeletal benefits beyond weight loss with a particular emphasis on the reduction in progression of osteoarthritis and inflammatory arthritis.

In our trauma section, Cosgrove and Sallade discuss synthetic electrospun fiber materials and their versatility for soft tissue management in orthopedic trauma. They report clinical evidence demonstrating improved wound healing and low complications in both topical and subdermal use in open fractures, degloving injuries, Achilles repairs, and amputations. Raszka and colleagues discuss transverse tibial transport for limb salvage in ischemic lower-extremity injuries. They report that this technique combined with endovascular therapy significantly improves amputation-free survival with minor complications.

Barré and Kluck discuss how distraction osteogenesis continues to evolve within the expanding field of regenerative medicine in pediatric orthopedics. This technique harnesses the biologic response to controlled mechanical stimulation

Orthop Clin N Am 57 (2026) xi–xii
https://doi.org/10.1016/j.ocl.2026.07.001
0030-5898/26/© 2026 Published by Elsevier Inc.

and enables the formation of native, vascularized bone and soft tissue. They review the basic principles, perioperative factors, and contemporary strategies for pediatric limb lengthening.

Foot and ankle tendinopathies are common problems with a "treatment gap" between surgery and conservative management that orthobiologics have the potential to fill. Quirolgico and colleagues provide an overview of the most commonly used orthobiologics and their use in the treatment of foot and ankle tendinopathies.

We thank the authors for their valuable contributions to the literature and hope that readers will find these reviews helpful in their practices.

Frederick M. Azar, MD
Department of Orthopaedic Surgery and Biomedical Engineering
Campbell Clinic
University of Tennessee-Campbell Clinic
1211 Union Avenue, Suite 510
Memphis, TN 38104, USA

E-mail address:
fazar@campbellclinic.com

Knee and Hip

Osteoarthritis as a Whole-Joint Disease, Part I: Current Standard of Care and Structural Therapeutic Targets in Cartilage, Synovium, and Subchondral Bone

Shlok V. Patel, MD[a], Kathleen Derwin, PhD[b], Xiaojuan Li, PhD[b,c], Suneel S. Apte, MBBS, DPhil[b], Nicolas S. Piuzzi, MD[a,b,*]

KEYWORDS

• Osteoarthritis • Disease-modifying osteoarthritis drug (DMOAD) • Therapeutic targets
• Phenotype • Endotype

KEY POINTS

- Guideline-supported conservative osteoarthritis care remains centered on patient education, exercise, weight optimization, NSAIDs, and short-term intra-articular corticosteroid use.
- No approved disease-modifying osteoarthritis drug is currently available; most existing treatments remain symptom-directed.
- Emerging structural therapeutic strategies have shown biological and imaging signals, but durable clinical benefit has been inconsistent, underscoring the need for phenotype-informed trial design and better alignment between structural and patient-reported endpoints.

INTRODUCTION

Osteoarthritis (OA), most often involving the hip, knee, and hand, is the most common type of arthritis and remains a major driver of chronic pain and long-term disability in adults.[1,2] It imposes a substantial economic burden, amounting to about $80 billion in US health care spending in 2016.[3,4] Historically, OA was viewed largely as a "wear-and-tear" consequence of aging and mechanical overload, with cartilage degeneration considered the primary pathologic feature. However, accumulating evidence now supports OA as a complex, whole-joint disorder involving not only cartilage, but also subchondral bone, synovium, ligaments, menisci, and periarticular muscle, with inflammatory and metabolic pathways contributing to symptom burden and structural progression.[5,6]

Contemporary OA care remains anchored in guideline-endorsed non-pharmacological "core" management consisting of patient education, exercise/rehabilitation, and weight optimization, supplemented by symptom-directed therapies such as topical/oral non-steroidal anti-inflammatory drugs (NSAIDs) and intra-articular injections, with total joint arthroplasty reserved for end-stage disease.[7,8] However, these strategies are

[a] Department of Orthopaedic Surgery, Cleveland Clinic, Cleveland, OH, USA; [b] Department of Biomedical Engineering, Lerner Research Institute, Cleveland Clinic, Cleveland, OH, USA; [c] Program for Advanced Musculoskeletal Imaging, Cleveland Clinic, Cleveland, OH, USA
* Corresponding author. Department of Orthopaedic Surgery, Cleveland Clinic, 9500 Euclid Avenue, A41, Cleveland, OH 44195.
E-mail address: piuzzin@ccf.org

Orthop Clin N Am 57 (2026) 277–287
https://doi.org/10.1016/j.ocl.2026.05.001

Abbreviations	
BML	bone marrow lesion
DMOAD	disease–modifying osteoarthritis drug
ECM	extracellular matrix
FGF	fibroblast growth factor
IL	Interleukin
MEPE	matrix extracellular phosphoglycoprotein
MMP	matrix metalloproteinase
NSAID	non–steroidal anti–inflammatory drug
OA	osteoarthritis
TGF–β	transforming growth factor–β
TG–C	TissueGene–C

largely palliative, and the field still lacks a durable, broadly applicable disease-modifying therapy that meets regulatory thresholds for clinically meaningful benefit while maintaining acceptable long-term safety. Although preclinical and early-phase clinical studies have been promising, phase 3 trials have not yielded consistent success, and no disease-modifying osteoarthritis drug (DMOAD) is currently approved or widely available.[9,10]

These setbacks may, in part, reflect the marked heterogeneity of OA potentially attributable to diverse etiologies, indolence and chronic, phasic nature. Rather than a single uniform disease process, OA manifests through diverse clinical patterns that vary in structural involvement, symptom burden, biomechanics, metabolic milieu, and pain processing,[11] which furthermore, may vary from joint to joint. In turn, this variability likely reflects differing contributions of biological pathways acting within, as well as across cartilage, synovium, subchondral bone, periarticular tissues, and systemic networks. This recognition has shifted the field toward clinical phenotype-enriched trial designs and more mechanism-informed therapeutic development, with the aim of improving signal detection and accelerating the development of effective disease-modifying strategies.[9] In this review, the first of a two-part series, we examine current and emerging therapeutic targets (**Fig. 1**, **Table 1**), spanning cartilage-directed agents, inflammation and synovitis-targeted approaches, and subchondral bone agents. Other emerging therapeutic strategies, including pain pathway modulation, metabolic interventions, senescence-directed therapies, orthobiologics, and drug delivery, are addressed in a companion review.

CURRENT STANDARD-OF-CARE

Current guidelines endorse a multimodal, patient-centered strategy grounded in shared decision-making and individualized risk–benefit assessment.[8] For both knee and hip OA, strongly recommended foundational therapies include structured exercise (eg, aerobic walking, strengthening, neuromuscular and aquatic programs), weight loss for overweight or obese patients and self-management/self-efficacy programs. Tai chi and cane use are also strongly recommended when clinically indicated. For symptom control, the guideline strongly recommends oral NSAIDs as first-line oral pharmacotherapy and intra-articular glucocorticoid injections for short-term pain relief; for hip injections, ultrasound guided injection is strongly recommended. For knee OA, topical NSAIDs and tibiofemoral bracing are additionally strongly recommended.[8,12]

Several modalities are conditionally recommended, reflecting lower-certainty evidence and the importance of tailoring to patient priorities and contraindications. For knee and hip OA, these include balance exercises, cognitive behavioral therapy, acupuncture, and local heat or cold; acetaminophen, duloxetine, and tramadol are conditionally recommended as alternatives when NSAIDs are inappropriate or inadequate. Knee-specific conditional options include yoga, patellofemoral bracing, radiofrequency ablation, topical capsaicin, and kinesiotaping.

The ACR/AF guideline recommends against multiple commonly used interventions because of limited efficacy and/or safety and standardization concerns, including glucosamine and chondroitin sulfate, bisphosphonates, hydroxychloroquine, methotrexate, platelet-rich plasma and stem cell injections, and biological agents.[8,12] Expert guidelines, such as those from OARSI and ACR/AF, strongly advise against both platelet-rich plasma and stem cell therapies due to extremely low-quality evidence, significant clinical heterogeneity, and a lack of standardization in how these biological formulations are prepared.[8,13] Similarly, use of intra-articular hyaluronic acid (hyaluronan;HA) injections remains controversial; the AAOS, NICE, and ACR/AF guidelines advise against their routine use citing inconsistent evidence and limited clinical benefit compared with saline.[8,12,14] Consequently, professional societies

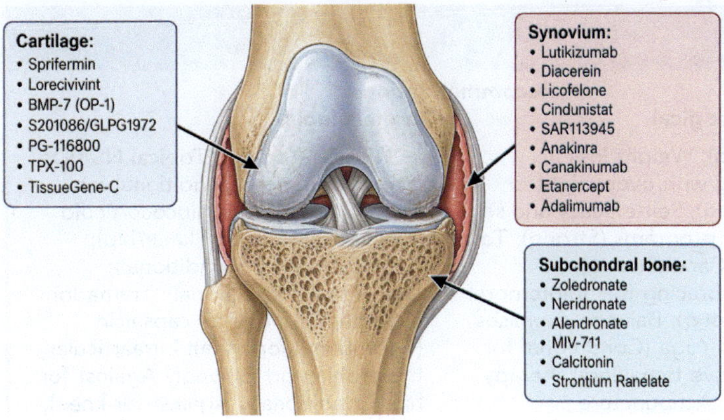

Fig. 1. Tissue-specific mechanisms of next-generation DMOADs. Schematic overview of the therapeutic targets discussed in this review. DMOAD, disease-modifying osteoarthritis drug.

caution against the routine clinical use of these regenerative therapies outside of carefully designed trials. In contrast to these alternatives, intra-articular corticosteroid injections are consistently endorsed across all major guidelines to provide acute, short-term pain relief (typically lasting between 2 and 12 weeks).[14] They are particularly recommended when other pharmacological therapies are unsuitable or ineffective, or to support patient participation in therapeutic exercise. The following table summarizes the current OA management guidelines (Table 2).

WHOLE-JOINT OSTEOARTHRITIS PHENOTYPES, MECHANISTIC PATHWAYS, AND THERAPEUTIC TARGETS

OA is best understood not as a single therapeutic problem, but as a set of interacting tissue-level and systemic processes that may each offer distinct opportunities for intervention. Each of the phenotypic and biological axes described in the introduction represents a distinct therapeutic entry point for disease modification. The subsections below examine the major tissue-level domains: cartilage, synovium, and subchondral

Table 1
Overview of novel DMOADs

Drug	Therapeutic Category	Tissue Targeted	Mechanism of Action	Signal
Lorecivivint (SM04690)	Wnt/β-catenin pathway modulation	Cartilage	Small-molecule CLK/DYRK inhibitor; modulates Wnt signaling to favor chondrogenesis	Mixed
Sprifermin	FGF-18 analog	Cartilage	Recombinant FGF-18; promotes chondrocyte proliferation and matrix production	Mixed
TissueGene-C (TG-C)	Cell + Gene Therapy	Cartilage	Allogeneic chondrocytes expressing TGF-β1; local anabolic delivery	Mixed
MIV-711	Cathepsin K inhibitor	Subchondral bone	Selective Cathepsin K inhibitor; reduces subchondral bone remodeling	Mixed
S201086 (GLPG1972)	ADAMTS Inhibitors	Cartilage	Aggrecanase inhibitor; aims to stop cartilage catabolism	Negative
TPX-100	MEPE analog	Cartilage	23-amino acid peptide derived from MEPE; promotes cartilage repair	Mixed
Lutikizumab (ABT-981)	Interleukin inhibitor	Synovium/ Inflammation	Dual variable domain immunoglobulin neutralizing IL-1 alpha and IL-1 beta	Negative
Cindunistat (SD-6010)	iNOS inhibitor	Synovium/ Inflammation	Irreversible inhibitor of human inducible nitric oxide synthase	Negative

Table 2
Guidelines for management of OA

Organization	Year	Recommendations: Non-pharmacological	Recommendations: Pharmacologic
ACR/AF[a]	2019	Exercise (Strong); Weight loss in patients living with overweight or obesity (Strong); Self-efficacy and self-management programs (Strong); Tai chi (Strong); Cane (Strong); Tibiofemoral bracing for tibiofemoral knee OA (Strong); Balance exercises (Conditional); Yoga (Conditional for knee); Cognitive behavioral therapy (Conditional); Acupuncture (Conditional); Thermal modalities (Conditional); Manual therapy (Conditionally Against); TENS (Strongly Against)	Oral NSAIDs (Strong); Topical NSAIDs (Strong for knee, Conditional for hand); Intraarticular glucocorticoid injections (Strong for knee/hip); Acetaminophen (Conditional); Duloxetine (Conditional); Tramadol (Conditional); Topical capsaicin (Conditional for knee); Intraarticular hyaluronic acid (Strongly Against for hip, Conditionally Against for knee); Non-tramadol opioids (Conditionally Against)
AAOS[b]	2021	Supervised, unsupervised, or aquatic exercise (Strong); Self-management programs (Strong); Patient education (Strong); Neuromuscular training (Moderate); Sustained weight loss (Moderate); Canes (Moderate); Braces (Moderate); Manual therapy (Limited); Massage (Limited); Acupuncture (Limited); TENS (Limited); Laser treatment (Limited); Extracorporeal shockwave therapy (Limited); Lateral wedge insoles (Strongly Not Recommended)	Oral NSAIDs (Strong); Oral Acetaminophen (Strong); Intra-articular Corticosteroids (Moderate); Topical NSAIDs (Strong); Intra-articular Hyaluronic Acid (Moderately Not Recommended); Platelet-rich Plasma (Limited); Oral Narcotics/Tramadol (Strongly Not Recommended)
NICE[c]	2022	Therapeutic exercise (Offer); Weight management (Offer); Walking aids (Consider); Supervised exercise (Consider); Manual therapy alongside exercise for hip/knee (Consider); Acupuncture or dry needling (Do not offer); TENS, ultrasound, or laser (Do not offer); Routine insoles, braces, or tape (Do not routinely offer)	Topical NSAIDs for knee (Offer); Oral NSAIDs with gastroprotection (Consider); Paracetamol or weak opioids (Do not routinely offer); Intra-articular corticosteroid injections (Consider); Intra-articular hyaluronan (Do not offer); Glucosamine (Do not offer); Strong opioids (Do not offer)
OARSI[d]	2019	Arthritis education (Core); Structured land-based exercise (Core); Dietary weight management (Core for knee); Mind-body exercise/Tai Chi/Yoga (Level 1B); Aquatic exercise (Level 1B/2 for knee); Gait aids (Level 1B/2); Cognitive behavioral therapy (Level 1B/2); Self-management programs (Level 1B/2)	Topical NSAIDs for knee (Level 1A); Oral NSAIDs - selective or non-selective + PPI (Level 1B for knee, Level 2 for hip); Intra-articular Corticosteroids (Level 1B/2); Intra-articular Hyaluronic Acid (Level 1B/2 for knee); Acetaminophen (Level 4A/4B- Conditionally Not Recommended); Oral/Transdermal Opioids (Level 5 - Strongly Not Recommended)

Abbreviations: AAOS, American Academy of Orthopaedic Surgeons; ACR/AF, American College of Rheumatology/Arthritis Foundation; NICE, National Institute for Health and Care Excellence; NSAID, non-steroidal anti-inflammatory drug; OARSI, Osteoarthritis Research Society International; PPI, proton pump inhibitor.

[a] ACR/AF: Recommendations are classified as Strong or Conditional, either for or against an intervention.

[b] AAOS: Recommendation strength is graded as Strong, Moderate, Limited, or Consensus.

[c] NICE: Recommendations are expressed using directive language rather than evidence grades: Offer, Consider, Do not offer, and Do not routinely offer.

[d] OARSI: Level 1A indicates ≥75% panel agreement with >50% strong recommendation in favor; Level 1B indicates ≥75% agreement with >50% conditional recommendation in favor; Level 2 indicates 60% to 74% agreement in favor. Levels 4A/4B indicate conditional recommendations against use, whereas Level 5 indicates a strong recommendation against use.

bone, and the emerging disease-modifying interventions targeting them.[9,11,15] Additional evolving strategies, including nociception-targeted approaches, metabolic interventions, senescence-directed therapies, orthobiologics, and other intra-articular regenerative treatments, are discussed in part-II of the review.

Cartilage-centric Therapies

Sprifermin, a recombinant human fibroblast growth factor (FGF) 18 remains the clearest proof-of-principle that cartilage structure can be modified in human OA using modern imaging. It has been investigated as a potential anabolic intra-articular DMOAD. In the FORWARD randomized trial (NCT01919164), intra-articular sprifermin 100 µg every 6 or 12 months produced a statistically significant increase in total femorotibial cartilage thickness at 2 years versus placebo, while WOMAC pain outcomes improved similarly across groups, highlighting uncertain clinical importance and durability.[16,17] Subsequent analyses have explored whether a "subgroup at risk" (more likely to progress structurally) may be more likely to show symptomatic separation over longer follow-up, reinforcing the broader lesson that cartilage-directed agents may require risk-based cohort selection and longer horizons to demonstrate efficacy or specify structural rather than symptomatic endpoints.

Transforming growth factor-β (TGF-β) signaling is central to cartilage homeostasis; physiologic loading activates latent TGF-β in articular cartilage, supporting the differentiated chondrocyte phenotype, suppressing hypertrophy, promoting lubricin expression, and dampening inflammatory signaling. In OA, however, active TGF-β levels are increased within the joint and can shift the signaling balance toward maladaptive responses that contribute to synovial fibrosis, osteophyte formation, and subchondral bone remodeling. This context-dependent biology means that both loss of baseline TGF-β signaling and excessive/redistributed activation can be deleterious, complicating therapeutic strategies that aim to either augment or inhibit the pathway.[18,19]

TissueGene-C (TG-C) is an intra-articular cell/gene therapy designed to deliver a localized anabolic signal via TGF-β1 overexpression, using a 3:1 cell mixture of non-transduced allogeneic human chondrocytes and genetically modified chondrocytes expressing TGF-β1 administered as a single intraarticular injection. Development began in South Korea, culminating in a 52 week phase III trial completed in 2015 that enrolled 163 patients with degenerative knee OA (NCT02072070) and demonstrated significant improvements in pain and function versus placebo, while directional trends toward greater cartilage thickness and slower subchondral bone changes were not statistically significant over the study period.[20] In the United States, TG-C has been studied in a multi-center, double-blind, placebo-controlled phase II trial in patients with moderate knee OA (NCT01221441).[21,22] At 12 months, a single intra-articular injection was associated with clinically meaningful improvements in patient-reported pain and function and with less MRI progression of whole-knee cartilage damage and synovitis features compared with placebo, without an apparent increase in adverse events; effects on osteophytes and other marrow lesion-type findings were not clearly different. TG-C is being evaluated in 2 ongoing US phase III trials (NCT03203330 and NCT03291470), with anticipated completion in 2025 and 2026, respectively.

Bone morphogenetic proteins (BMPs) are members of the TGF-β superfamily with key roles in skeletal development and cartilage homeostasis, which has made them attractive candidates for cartilage repair and disease modification in OA. In preclinical models, BMPs have been delivered using viral and non-viral gene constructs and scaffold-based composites, most commonly using BMP-2 as well as BMP-6, BMP-7, and BMP-9, with the goal of stimulating matrix synthesis and osteochondral regeneration.[23,24] Clinically, however, translation remains limited by uncertainty around optimal dosing, delivery strategy, and patient selection, and the existing human evidence is largely early phase. For instance, intra-articular BMP-7 (OP-1) has phase I data supporting feasibility and acceptable safety (including no clear signal of ectopic bone formation on radiographs), but has not yet produced definitive late-phase efficacy or structural outcomes.[25] Two randomized clinical trials (NCT01111045, NCT01133613) have been completed with results not publicly available, underscoring that the BMP field in OA remains biologically compelling but not yet clinically validated.

Wnt/β-catenin pathway modulation (lorecivivint/SM04690) targets chondrocyte and joint-tissue transcriptional pathways implicated in OA progression.[7,10] Lorecivivint is an intra-articular small molecule that inhibits the kinases CLK2 and DYRK1A and modulates Wnt pathway signaling. In a phase 2b trial (NCT03122860), 0.07 and 0.23 mg doses of intraarticular lorecivivint in the more painful knee demonstrated significant improvements in WOMAC pain and function over 24 weeks, supporting continued development and, importantly, fueling the rationale for phenotype -directed evaluation.[26] Several phase III trials have completed in the past 2 to 3 years with results not yet reported (NCT05603754, NCT03928184, NCT04385303, NCT04520607, NCT05603754).[10] Another Wnt pathway inhibitor, XAV-939, has been shown in experimental traumatic OA models to attenuate disease severity, with proposed mechanisms that include reduced chondrocyte catabolic activity and suppression of fibrotic responses in synovial fibroblasts.[27]

Extracellular matrix (ECM) is responsible for the unique mechanical attributes of cartilage and targeting its breakdown has been an important and consistently explored therapeutic angle. ADAMTS-5 inhibition or blockade is one of the most biologically compelling anti-catabolic strategies.[23,28,29] ADAMTS-5 is a principal secreted protease that cleaves aggrecan, a major cartilage extracellular matrix proteoglycan, and may therefore drive early cartilage matrix loss in OA.[30,31] However, the ROCCELLA phase 2 trial using an ADAMTS5 inhibitor, S201086/GLPG1972 did not demonstrate significant differences versus placebo in MRI-assessed cartilage loss in the central medial femorotibial compartment at 52 weeks, nor in key symptomatic endpoints.[32] However, since the study participants had established knee OA Kellgren-Lawrence grade 2 or 3 and Osteoarthritis Research Society International joint space narrowing (grade 1 or 2), it is possible that there was a disconnect with the putative biological action of ADAMTS5 in early cartilage loss, illustrating the translational challenge of aligning target biology with human OA, especially given the lack of biomarkers for early OA.

Matrix metalloproteinases (MMPs), like ADAMTS5, are zinc-dependent secreted and cell-surface proteases that have a prominent role in ECM turnover. In OA, they are believed to be central to irreversible collagen degradation, with MMP-13 receiving particular focus because of its strong activity against type II collagen and its upregulation in degenerating cartilage.[7,33] Broad-spectrum MMP inhibition has not translated into effective OA therapy. A large 12 month randomized trial of the broad-spectrum oral MMP inhibitor PG-116800 showed no benefit in radiographic joint space width or WOMAC outcomes and was limited by musculoskeletal toxicity.[33] Current work has therefore shifted toward selective MMP-13 inhibition using non-zinc-binding/allosteric designs to improve specificity and reduce toxicity.[34,35] In parallel, local delivery strategies are emerging, including enzyme-responsive injectable platforms that release an MMP-13 blocker in situ and attenuate cartilage degeneration in preclinical OA models.[36]

TPX-100 is an intra-articular synthetic peptide derived from matrix extracellular phosphoglycoprotein (MEPE), a protein linked to osteochondral homeostasis that appears reduced in arthritic tissue.[37] In a phase II study (NCT01925261), weekly intra-articular dosing was generally well tolerated, and although the prespecified MRI endpoint of cartilage thickness did not show clear separation at 6 to 12 months in the main efficacy cohort, patient-reported outcomes (WOMAC/KOOS domains) favored TPX-100-treated knees in reported analyses. Importantly, a retrospective MRI analysis using 3D femoral bone shape suggested that TPX-100 was associated with less pathologic bone shape change at 6 and 12 months vs placebo knees, a finding interpreted as potentially relevant to downstream joint failure risk.[38] Consistent with that trajectory, newer clinical development has emphasized bone-shape-based selection/assessment, reflecting a strategic pivot toward osteochondral biomarkers as candidate surrogates for DMOAD development.[39]

Synovitis/Inflammation-targeted Therapies

Efforts to treat knee and hip OA by directly suppressing synovial inflammation have largely not reproduced the "plug-and-play" success seen in inflammatory arthritides, in part because OA synovitis is often low-grade, heterogeneous, and variably coupled to pain/structure. Oral/topical NSAIDs and selective COX-2 inhibitors reduce prostaglandin-driven nociceptor sensitization and synovial inflammatory tone and remain the most consistently effective pharmacological option for symptomatic inflammatory flares but have no consistent disease-modifying signal.[7,37,40] Intra-articular corticosteroids can provide short-term relief in inflammatory flares with well-known limitations for durability and repeated exposure.[2,7,41,42] Dual Interleukin (IL)-1α/β inhibition via lutikizumab has been evaluated in knee OA. In a randomized phase 1 multiple-dose knee OA study (NCT01668511; $n = 36$), ABT-981 was generally tolerated and showed pharmacodynamic target engagement (reductions in circulating IL-1α/β and inflammatory/tissue-turnover biomarkers).[43] The key efficacy test was the phase II synovitis-enriched ILLUSTRATE-K trial (NCT02087904; KL 2–3; $n = 350$), in which 25/100/200 mg SC every 2 weeks for 50 weeks produced only a borderline, transient WOMAC pain improvement at week 16 with 100 mg ($P = .050$) and no improvement in MRI-assessed synovitis or other key symptom/structural outcomes at later time points; injection-site reactions and neutropenia-related discontinuations were more frequent than placebo.[44] Collectively, these data suggest that while IL-1 blockade can achieve biological suppression, it has not translated into durable clinical benefit in knee OA, supporting future strategies that refine inflammatory endotyping selection or pursue upstream innate circuit modulation rather than standalone IL-1 neutralization.

Symptomatic slow-acting anti-inflammatory agents with putative structure effects have produced mixed results: diacerein (IL-1 modulation, anti-catabolic/pro-anabolic properties in preclinical models) showed reduced radiographic joint space narrowing over 3 years in hip OA in a placebo-controlled trial (ECHODIAH), but real-world uptake has been constrained by tolerability/safety considerations and heterogeneity in downstream studies.[45] Licofelone (dual 5-lipoxygenase/COX inhibitor) achieved symptom improvement comparable to naproxen in knee OA, with quantitative MRI suggesting slower cartilage volume loss, illustrating how anti-inflammatory pathway selection plus sensitive imaging endpoints can reveal signals that radiographs often miss.[46–48] By contrast, several downstream inflammatory pathway inhibitors have disappointed in large trials: the iNOS inhibitor cindunistat (SD-6010) did not slow knee OA joint space narrowing or pain overall, with only transient, non-sustained subgroup signals, and intra-articular IKK/NF-κB pathway inhibition (SAR113945) did not improve WOMAC pain in the overall phase 2 study population, with only post hoc suggestions of benefit in effusion-enriched subsets.[10,49,50] Collectively, findings reinforce that broad suppression of inflammatory mediators in unselected OA rarely translates into durable clinical impact.

Among biologics, TNF inhibition has produced inconsistent and generally non-definitive signals in knee OA: small studies of intra-articular etanercept and adalimumab reported short-term pain improvements, but these designs and sizes limit inference about durable efficacy or imaging/structural effects.[51,52] Intra-articular anakinra was well tolerated but did not improve WOMAC scores vs placebo in knee OA.[53] Even systemic inflammation may matter for a subset: exploratory analyses from CANTOS RCT found fewer incident hip and knee replacements with canakinumab, indirectly supporting an "inflammation-responsive" subgroup hypothesis.[54] Some "inflammation-targeting" approaches show context-dependent promise: oral methotrexate improved knee pain and function at 6 months in a UK multicenter RCT, yet a separate MRI effusion-synovitis–enriched knee OA RCT found no improvement in pain or synovitis over 52 weeks, highlighting how enrollment criteria and endpoints may affect study outcomes.[55,56]

Subchondral Bone-targeted Therapies

Subchondral bone is an active participant in OA. Early OA can feature increased bone turnover, microdamage, angiogenesis, and remodeling that alters load transfer to cartilage. Bone marrow lesions (BMLs) on MRI reflect a composite of edema-like changes, fibrosis, necrosis, and remodeling, and have been repeatedly linked to pain fluctuation and structural deterioration in OA subsets, making them a biologically coherent enrichment feature for bone-targeted trials.[7,10,57]

Early proof-of-concept work suggested that a single zoledronic acid 5 mg infusion could reduce knee pain and BML size over short-term follow-up in patients selected for BMLs, but these signals did not translate into consistent disease-modifying benefit in a larger multicenter ZAP2 RCT: 2 annual zoledronic acid infusions did not slow tibiofemoral cartilage volume loss and did not improve pain or BML size versus placebo over 24 months.[58,59] Where bisphosphonates may retain clinical value is in mechanistically enriched scenarios: for instance, in acute painful knee OA with MRI-confirmed BMLs, intravenous neridronate improved pain and reduced BML size over short follow-up, supporting a lesion-targeted analgesic/anti-remodeling concept rather than a universal OA strategy.[60] In hip OA, a 2 year randomized study of weekly alendronate reported symptomatic improvement without clear prevention of structural progression, reinforcing that symptom and structure can dissociate and that patient selection is likely decisive.[61] Consistent with this heterogeneity, meta-analyses have reached divergent conclusions overall, with some suggesting little to no average benefit in unselected knee OA populations, further underscoring that any clinical utility is most plausible in high–bone-turnover/BML-predominant presentations rather than routine OA care.[62]

MIV-711 is an oral, selective cathepsin K inhibitor designed to modulate the osteochondral unit by suppressing osteoclast-mediated collagen degradation and downstream bone remodeling signals that can accelerate cartilage loss.[10] In a randomized, double-blind phase IIa trial ($n = 244$; Kellgren-Lawrence grade 2–3), participants received placebo or oral MIV-711

(100 or 200 mg) once daily for 26 weeks. Although MIV-711 did not significantly improve pain versus placebo, it showed evidence of a structural signal on MRI, with reduced progression of medial femoral subchondral bone area (both doses) and less medial femoral cartilage thinning (most consistently with 100 mg), with a generally reassuring safety profile over the treatment period.[63]

Other bone-cartilage axis therapies have provided important proof-of-concept but limited near-term clinical uptake. In two phase 3 trials, oral salmon calcitonin did not demonstrate a statistically significant benefit on radiographic joint space narrowing at 24 months, despite reported improvements in WOMAC outcomes and bone/joint turnover biomarkers.[64] As such, calcitonin does not yet have an established and clear clinical role as a DMOAD in knee OA. Among bone-targeted agents, strontium ranelate has shown the clearest evidence of structural benefit: in the 3 year SEKOIA trial, strontium ranelate was associated with less joint space width loss than placebo, with modest symptomatic improvement.[65] MRI-focused analyses also suggested benefits on cartilage volume loss and BML progression in subsets.[66] However, its OA relevance has remained largely academic because regulatory restrictions driven by cardiovascular and venous thromboembolism risk sharply limit its use.[67]

SUMMARY

Across the 3 structural axes that define the intra-articular target space in OA—cartilage, synovium, and subchondral bone—several drug candidates have produced biologically coherent, and at times statistically significant, structural signals on quantitative MRI or radiography. Few, however, appear to have translated these signals into durable, clinically meaningful patient-reported benefit in unselected populations. A recurring lesson from phase 2 and 3 programs is that patient selection and trial design may matter as much as target biology itself. Broad enrollment and short follow-up have often seemed insufficient to demonstrate a credible disease-modifying effect, whereas enrichment for structural, inflammatory, or bone-remodeling phenotypes may offer a more promising path. Addressing OA as a whole-joint disease, however, likely requires extending this framework beyond the joint itself. In the companion review, we examine therapeutic targets in pain-processing pathways, systemic metabolic biology, and aging-related mechanisms, alongside contemporary intra-articular regenerative strategies, and discuss the infrastructure, biomarker, and trial-design reforms that may help translate mechanistic insight into more durable, phenotype-matched care.

CLINICS CARE POINTS

- Beyond "One-Size-Fits-All": OA is a heterogeneous condition that requires individualized management. Treatment strategies must align with the patient's dominant clinical phenotype, symptom burden, functional limitations, and relevant comorbidities. Optimal care also demands consideration of the underlying molecular endotypes driving the disease.
- The Foundation is Non-Negotiable: Structured exercise, patient education, and weight optimization remain the high-certainty core of management for all patients, regardless of radiographic severity.
- Bridge the Structure-Symptom Gap: Structural improvements on an MRI (such as increased cartilage thickness) are biological triumphs but perception of symptomatic improvement is a necessary accompanying metric of success. Future disease-modifying therapies must be judged by their ability to translate structural stability into meaningful improvements in PROMs.

DISCLOSURES

N.S. Piuzzi has the following disclosures not related to the present study: Grants or contracts—Osteal Therapeutics, Peptilogics, RegenLab, Signature Orthopedics, Zimmer, and Stryker; Consulting fees—Zimmer, Pacira Pharmaceutical, and Stryker; Editorial board member or Leadership role—*JBJS, American Association of Hip and Knee Surgeons, and Orthopaedic Research Society*. All the other authors have no disclosures.

REFERENCES

1. Lespasio MJ, Sultan AA, Piuzzi NS, et al. Hip osteoarthritis: a primer. Perm J 2018;22(1):17–084.
2. Lespasio MJ, Piuzzi NS, Husni ME, et al. Knee osteoarthritis: a primer. Perm J 2017;21:16–183. PubMed PMID: 29035179; PubMed Central PMCID: PMC5638628.
3. Dieleman JL, Baral R, Birger M, et al. US spending on personal health care and public health, 1996-2013. JAMA 2016;316(24):2627–46. PubMed PMID: 28027366; PubMed Central PMCID: PMC 5551483.
4. GBD 2021 Osteoarthritis Collaborators. Global, regional, and national burden of osteoarthritis,

1990-2020 and projections to 2050: a systematic analysis for the global burden of disease study 2021. Lancet Rheumatol 2023;5(9):e508–22. https://doi.org/10.1016/S2665-9913(23)00163-7. PubMed PMID: 37675071; PubMed Central PMCID: PMC10477960.
5. Loeser RF, Goldring SR, Scanzello CR, et al. Osteoarthritis: a disease of the joint as an organ. Arthritis Rheum 2012;64(6):1697–707. PubMed PMID: 22392533; PubMed Central PMCID: PMC3366018.
6. Hunter DJ, Bierma-Zeinstra S. Osteoarthritis. Lancet 2019;393(10182):1745–59.
7. Cho Y, Jeong S, Kim H, et al. Disease-modifying therapeutic strategies in osteoarthritis: current status and future directions. Exp Mol Med 2021;53(11):1689–96. PubMed PMID: 34848838; PubMed Central PMCID: PMC8640059.
8. Kolasinski SL, Neogi T, Hochberg MC, et al. 2019 American College of Rheumatology/Arthritis Foundation Guideline for the management of osteoarthritis of the hand, hip, and knee. Arthritis Care Res 2020;72(2):149–62. PubMed PMID: 31908149; PubMed Central PMCID: PMC11488261.
9. Van Spil WE, Kubassova O, Boesen M, et al. Osteoarthritis phenotypes and novel therapeutic targets. Biochem Pharmacol 2019;165:41–8. Therapeutic Advances in Arthritis Diseases.
10. Brandt MD, Malone JB, Kean TJ. Advances and challenges in the pursuit of disease-modifying osteoarthritis drugs: a review of 2010–2024 clinical trials. Biomedicines 2025;13(2). https://doi.org/10.3390/biomedicines13020355.
11. Mantripragada VP, Csorba A, Bova W, et al. Assessment of clinical, tissue, and cell-level metrics identify four biologically distinct knee osteoarthritis patient phenotypes. Cartilage 2022;13(1):19476035221074003. https://doi.org/10.1177/19476035221074003. PubMed PMID: 35109693; PubMed Central PMCID: PMC9137310.
12. Brophy RH, Fillingham YA. AAOS Clinical Practice Guideline summary: management of osteoarthritis of the knee (Nonarthroplasty), third edition. J Am Acad Orthop Surg 2022;30(9):e721–9.
13. Bannuru RR, Osani MC, Vaysbrot EE, et al. OARSI guidelines for the non-surgical management of knee, hip, and polyarticular osteoarthritis. Osteoarthr Cartil 2019;27(11):1578–89.
14. Osteoarthritis in over 16s: diagnosis and management [Internet]. London: National Institute for Health and Care Excellence (NICE); 2022 [cited 2026 Apr 22]. (National Institute for Health and Care Excellence: Guidelines). Available at: http://www.ncbi.nlm.nih.gov/books/NBK588843/PubMed PMID:36745715.
15. Cao Y, Tang S, Ding C. Inflammatory phenotype of osteoarthritis and its potential therapies. Rheumatol Autoimmun 2021;1(2):92–100.
16. Guehring H, Moreau F, Daelken B, et al. The effects of sprifermin on symptoms and structure in a subgroup at risk of progression in the FORWARD knee osteoarthritis trial. Semin Arthritis Rheum 2021;51(2):450–6.
17. Hochberg MC, Guermazi A, Guehring H, et al. Effect of intra-articular sprifermin vs placebo on femorotibial joint cartilage thickness in patients with osteoarthritis. JAMA 2019;322(14):1360–70. PubMed PMID: 31593273; PubMed Central PMCID: PMC6784851.
18. van der Kraan PM, Goumans MJ, Blaney Davidson E, et al. Age-dependent alteration of TGF-β signalling in osteoarthritis. Cell Tissue Res 2012;347(1):257–65.
19. van der Kraan PM. Inhibition of transforming growth factor-β in osteoarthritis. Discrepancy with reduced TGFβ signaling in normal joints. Osteoarthr Cartil Open 2022;4(1):100238. https://doi.org/10.1016/j.ocarto.2022.100238. PubMed PMID: 36474474; PubMed Central PMCID: PMC9718219.
20. Kim MK, Ha CW, In Y, et al. A multicenter, double-blind, phase III clinical trial to evaluate the efficacy and safety of a cell and gene therapy in knee osteoarthritis patients. Hum Gene Ther Clin Dev 2018;29(1):48–59.
21. Guermazi A, Kalsi G, Niu J, et al. Structural effects of intra-articular TGF-β1 in moderate to advanced knee osteoarthritis: MRI-based assessment in a randomized controlled trial. BMC Muscoskelet Disord 2017;18(1):461. PubMed PMID: 29145839; PubMed Central PMCID: PMC5689208.
22. Lee B, Parvizi J, Bramlet D, et al. Results of a phase II study to determine the efficacy and safety of genetically engineered allogeneic human chondrocytes expressing TGF-β1. J Knee Surg 2020;33(2):167–72.
23. Zhu Z, Li J, Ruan G, et al. Investigational drugs for the treatment of osteoarthritis, an update on recent developments. Expert Opin Invest Drugs 2018;27(11):881–900.
24. Hayashi M, Muneta T, Ju YJ, et al. Weekly intra-articular injections of bone morphogenetic protein-7 inhibits osteoarthritis progression. Arthritis Res Ther 2008;10(5):R118. https://doi.org/10.1186/ar2521.
25. Hunter DJ, Pike MC, Jonas BL, et al. Phase 1 safety and tolerability study of BMP-7 in symptomatic knee osteoarthritis. BMC Muscoskelet Disord 2010;11:232. PubMed PMID: 20932341; PubMed Central PMCID: PMC2958989.
26. Yazici Y, McAlindon TE, Gibofsky A, et al. A phase 2b randomized trial of lorecivivint, a novel intra-articular CLK2/DYRK1A inhibitor and Wnt pathway modulator for knee osteoarthritis. Osteoarthr Cartil 2021;29(5):654–66.
27. Lietman C, Wu B, Lechner S, et al. Inhibition of Wnt/β-catenin signaling ameliorates osteoarthritis

in a murine model of experimental osteoarthritis. JCI Insight 2018;3(3):e96308. 96308.
28. Oo WM, Hunter DJ. Repurposed and investigational disease-modifying drugs in osteoarthritis (DMOADs). Ther Adv Musculoskelet Dis 2022;14: 1759720X221090297. https://doi.org/10.1177/1759720X221090297.
29. Apte SS. Anti-ADAMTS5 monoclonal antibodies: implications for aggrecanase inhibition in osteoarthritis. Biochem J 2016;473(1):e1–4. PubMed PMID: 26657033; PubMed Central PMCID: PMC5525052.
30. Abbaszade I, Liu RQ, Yang F, et al. Cloning and characterization of ADAMTS11, an aggrecanase from the ADAMTS family. J Biol Chem 1999;274-(33):23443–50.
31. Bhutada S, Hoyle A, Piuzzi NS, et al. Degradomics defines proteolysis information flow from human knee osteoarthritis cartilage to matched synovial fluid and the contributions of secreted proteases ADAMTS5, MMP13 and CMA1 to articular cartilage breakdown. Osteoarthr Cartil 2025;33(1):116–27. PubMed PMID: 39293776; PubMed Central PMCID: PMC12342059.
32. Schnitzer T, Pueyo M, Deckx H, et al. Evaluation of S201086/GLPG1972, an ADAMTS-5 inhibitor, for the treatment of knee osteoarthritis in ROCCELLA: a phase 2 randomized clinical trial. Osteoarthr Cartil 2023;31(7):985–94.
33. Krzeski P, Buckland-Wright C, Bálint G, et al. Development of musculoskeletal toxicity without clear benefit after administration of PG-116800, a matrix metalloproteinase inhibitor, to patients with knee osteoarthritis: a randomized, 12-month, double-blind, placebo-controlled study. Arthritis Res Ther 2007;9(5):R109. https://doi.org/10.1186/ar2315. PubMed PMID: 17958901; PubMed Central PMCID: PMC2212568.
34. Cuffaro D, Gimeno A, Bernardoni BL, et al. Identification of N-Acyl hydrazones as new non-zinc-binding MMP-13 inhibitors by structure-based virtual screening studies and chemical optimization. Int J Mol Sci 2023;24(13):11098. https://doi.org/10.3390/ijms241311098. PubMed PMID: 37446276; PubMed Central PMCID: PMC10342305.
35. Bendele AM, Neelagiri M, Neelagiri V, et al. Development of a selective matrix metalloproteinase 13 (MMP-13) inhibitor for the treatment of osteoarthritis. Eur J Med Chem 2021;224:113666. https://doi.org/10.1016/j.ejmech.2021.113666. PubMed PMID: 34245949; PubMed Central PMCID: PMC8511113.
36. Roy HS, Murugesan P, Kulkarni C, et al. On-demand release of a selective MMP-13 blocker from an enzyme-responsive injectable hydrogel protects cartilage from degenerative progression in osteoarthritis. J Mater Chem B 2024;12(22):5325–38.
37. Chen T, Weng W, Liu Y, et al. Update on novel non-operative treatment for osteoarthritis: current status and future trends. Front Pharmacol 2021;12: 755230. https://doi.org/10.3389/fphar.2021.755230. PubMed PMID: 34603064; PubMed Central PMCID: PMC8481638.
38. McGuire D, Bowes M, Brett A, et al. Study TPX-100-5: intra-articular TPX-100 significantly delays pathological bone shape change and stabilizes cartilage in moderate to severe bilateral knee OA. Arthritis Res Ther 2021;23(1):242. PubMed PMID: 34535197; PubMed Central PMCID: PMC8447757.
39. Brett AD, G Conaghan P. 3-dimensional bone shape and knee osteoarthritis: what have we learned? Osteoarthr Imaging 2024;4(1):100178. https://doi.org/10.1016/j.ostima.2024.100178.
40. Cai X, Yuan S, Zeng Y, et al. New trends in pharmacological treatments for osteoarthritis. Front Pharmacol 2021;12. https://doi.org/10.3389/fphar.2021.645842.
41. Grässel S, Muschter D. Recent advances in the treatment of osteoarthritis. F1000Res 2020;9. https://doi.org/10.12688/f1000research.22115.1. F1000 Faculty Rev-325.
42. McAlindon TE, LaValley MP, Harvey WF, et al. Effect of intra-articular triamcinolone vs saline on knee cartilage volume and pain in patients with knee osteoarthritis: a randomized clinical trial. JAMA 2017; 317(19):1967–75. PubMed PMID: 28510679; PubMed Central PMCID: PMC5815012.
43. Wang SX, Abramson SB, Attur M, et al. Safety, tolerability, and pharmacodynamics of an anti-interleukin-1α/β dual variable domain immunoglobulin in patients with osteoarthritis of the knee: a randomized phase 1 study. Osteoarthr Cartil 2017;25(12): 1952–61.
44. Fleischmann RM, Bliddal H, Blanco FJ, et al. A phase II trial of Lutikizumab, an Anti-Interleukin-1α/β dual variable domain immunoglobulin, in knee osteoarthritis patients with synovitis. Arthritis Rheumatol 2019;71(7):1056–69.
45. Dougados M, Nguyen M, Berdah L, et al. Evaluation of the structure-modifying effects of diacerein in hip osteoarthritis: ECHODIAH, a three-year, placebo-controlled trial. Evaluation of the chondromodulating effect of diacerein in OA of the hip. Arthritis Rheum 2001;44(11):2539–47, 2-t PubMed PMID: 11710710.
46. Raynauld JP, Martel-Pelletier J, Bias P, et al. Protective effects of licofelone, a 5-lipoxygenase and cyclo-oxygenase inhibitor, versus naproxen on cartilage loss in knee osteoarthritis: a first multicentre clinical trial using quantitative MRI. Ann Rheum Dis 2009;68(6):938–47.
47. Kulkarni SK, Singh VP. Licofelone: the answer to unmet needs in osteoarthritis therapy? Curr Rheumatol Rep 2008;10(1):43–8.
48. Pelletier JP, Boileau C, Boily M, et al. The protective effect of licofelone on experimental osteoarthritis is

correlated with the downregulation of gene expression and protein synthesis of several major cartilage catabolic factors: MMP-13, cathepsin K and aggrecanases. Arthritis Res Ther 2005;7(5):R1091–102. PubMed PMID: 16207326; PubMed Central PMCID: PMC1257437.
49. Hellio le Graverand MP, Clemmer RS, Redifer P, et al. A 2-year randomised, double-blind, placebo-controlled, multicentre study of oral selective iNOS inhibitor, cindunistat (SD-6010), in patients with symptomatic osteoarthritis of the knee. Ann Rheum Dis 2013;72(2):187–95.
50. Grothe K, Flechsenhar K, Paehler T, et al. IκB kinase inhibition as a potential treatment of osteoarthritis - results of a clinical proof-of-concept study. Osteoarthr Cartil 2017;25(1):46–52.
51. Ohtori S, Orita S, Yamauchi K, et al. Efficacy of direct injection of etanercept into knee joints for pain in moderate and severe knee osteoarthritis. Yonsei Med J 2015;56(5):1379–83. PubMed PMID: 26256983; PubMed Central PMCID: PMC4541670.
52. Wang J. Efficacy and safety of adalimumab by intra-articular injection for moderate to severe knee osteoarthritis: an open-label randomized controlled trial. J Int Med Res 2018;46(1):326–34. PubMed PMID: 28840750; PubMed Central PMCID: PMC6011328.
53. Chevalier X, Goupille P, Beaulieu AD, et al. Intraarticular injection of anakinra in osteoarthritis of the knee: a multicenter, randomized, double-blind, placebo-controlled study. Arthritis Rheum 2009; 61(3):344–52.
54. Schieker M, Conaghan PG, Mindeholm L, et al. Effects of Interleukin-1β inhibition on incident hip and knee replacement: exploratory analyses from a randomized, double-blind, placebo-controlled trial. Ann Intern Med 2020;173(7):509–15. PubMed PMID: 32744862; PubMed Central PMCID: PMC8503784.
55. Zhu Z, Yu Q, Leng X, et al. Low-dose methotrexate for the treatment of inflammatory knee osteoarthritis: a randomized clinical trial. JAMA Intern Med 2025;185(7):808–16. PubMed PMID: 40455462; PubMed Central PMCID: PMC12131170.
56. Kingsbury SR, Tharmanathan P, Keding A, et al. Pain reduction with oral methotrexate in knee osteoarthritis : a randomized, placebo-controlled clinical trial. Ann Intern Med 2024;177(9):1145–56.
57. Sundaram K, Vargas-Hernández JS, Sanchez TR, et al. Are subchondral intraosseous injections effective and safe for the treatment of knee osteoarthritis? A systematic review. J Knee Surg 2019; 32(11):1046–57.
58. Cai G, Aitken D, Laslett LL, et al. Effect of intravenous zoledronic acid on tibiofemoral cartilage volume among patients with knee osteoarthritis with bone marrow lesions: a randomized clinical trial. JAMA 2020;323(15):1456–66.
59. Laslett LL, Doré DA, Quinn SJ, et al. Zoledronic acid reduces knee pain and bone marrow lesions over 1 year: a randomised controlled trial. Ann Rheum Dis 2012;71(8):1322–8.
60. Varenna M, Zucchi F, Failoni S, et al. Intravenous neridronate in the treatment of acute painful knee osteoarthritis: a randomized controlled study. Rheumatology 2015;54(10):1826–32.
61. Nishii T, Tamura S, Shiomi T, et al. Alendronate treatment for hip osteoarthritis: prospective randomized 2-year trial. Clin Rheumatol 2013;32(12):1759–66.
62. Vaysbrot EE, Osani MC, Musetti MC, et al. Are bisphosphonates efficacious in knee osteoarthritis? A meta-analysis of randomized controlled trials. Osteoarthr Cartil 2018;26(2):154–64.
63. Conaghan PG, Bowes MA, Kingsbury SR, et al. Disease-modifying effects of a novel cathepsin k inhibitor in osteoarthritis: a randomized controlled trial. Ann Intern Med 2020;172(2):86–95.
64. Karsdal MA, Byrjalsen I, Alexandersen P, et al. Treatment of symptomatic knee osteoarthritis with oral salmon calcitonin: results from two phase 3 trials. Osteoarthr Cartil 2015;23(4):532–43.
65. Reginster JY, Badurski J, Bellamy N, et al. Efficacy and safety of strontium ranelate in the treatment of knee osteoarthritis: results of a double-blind, randomised placebo-controlled trial. Ann Rheum Dis 2013;72(2):179–86.
66. Pelletier JP, Roubille C, Raynauld JP, et al. Disease-modifying effect of strontium ranelate in a subset of patients from the phase III knee osteoarthritis study SEKOIA using quantitative MRI: reduction in bone marrow lesions protects against cartilage loss. Ann Rheum Dis 2015;74(2):422–9.
67. Reginster JY. Cardiac concerns associated with strontium ranelate. Expert Opin Drug Saf 2014; 13(9):1209–13. PubMed PMID: 25020233; PubMed Central PMCID: PMC4196504.

Osteoarthritis as a Whole-Joint Disease, Part II: Emerging Nociceptive, Metabolic, Senescence, and Regenerative Therapeutic Targets, with Perspectives on Precision Care

Shlok V. Patel, MD[a], Kathleen Derwin, PhD[b], Xiaojuan Li, PhD[b,c], Suneel S. Apte, MBBS, DPhil[b], Nicolas S. Piuzzi, MD[a,b,*]

KEYWORDS

• Osteoarthritis • Disease-modifying osteoarthritis drug (DMOAD) • Therapeutic targets • Phenotype • Endotype

KEY POINTS

- Osteoarthritis symptom burden and progression are influenced not only by intra-articular structural disease, but also by peripheral and central pain processing, systemic metabolic dysfunction, and aging-associated cellular senescence.
- Regenerative intra-articular therapies and drug-delivery innovations remain promising but unproven avenues for disease modification. Future progress will likely depend on better patient stratification, stronger biomarker and imaging end points, and delivery platforms that improve local durability and target engagement.
- Precision OA care will require moving beyond "one-size-fits-all" therapeutic trials toward phenotype- and endotype-enriched designs that integrate clinical features, imaging, biomarkers, omics, and predictive modeling to identify patients most likely to benefit.

INTRODUCTION

Osteoarthritis (OA) is the most common form of arthritis and a major cause of chronic pain and disability in adults, with a rising global burden and substantial health care costs.[1–4] Although cartilage degeneration has historically received the most attention, OA is now understood as a heterogeneous whole-joint disorder in which multiple tissues and systemic processes contribute to symptom burden and structural progression.[5,6] Current management remains centered on guideline-supported core strategies, including patient education, exercise, and weight optimization, with symptom-directed pharmacologic treatment and arthroplasty reserved for advanced disease. Despite ongoing therapeutic development, no disease-modifying OA is currently approved for routine use.[7–10]

[a] Department of Orthopaedic Surgery, Cleveland Clinic, Cleveland, OH, USA; [b] Department of Biomedical Engineering, Lerner Research Institute, Cleveland Clinic, Cleveland, OH, USA; [c] Program for Advanced Musculoskeletal Imaging, Cleveland Clinic, Cleveland, OH, USA
* Corresponding author. Department of Orthopaedic Surgery, Cleveland Clinic, 9500 Euclid Avenue, A41, Cleveland, OH 44195.
E-mail address: piuzzin@ccf.org

Orthop Clin N Am 57 (2026) 289–297
https://doi.org/10.1016/j.ocl.2026.05.002

Abbreviations	
HA	hyaluronic acid
NGF	nerve growth factor
OA	osteoarthritis
PRP	platelet-rich plasma
SASP	senescence-associated secretory phenotype

Recognition of OA heterogeneity has focused attention on phenotypes and endotypes as useful frameworks for therapeutic development.[11,12] Phenotypes describe observable patterns of disease, whereas endotypes refer to the biological mechanisms underlying those patterns. Although these constructs often overlap and remain incompletely resolved, they may help support patient stratification and more targeted therapeutic trial design in OA.[11] In the first part of this 2-part review, we examined the current standard of care and therapeutic targets within the joint compartment, including cartilage-directed agents, synovitis and inflammation modulators, and subchondral bone–acting therapies. In this second part, we address mechanism-based therapeutic targets that act outside the cartilage–synovium–bone axis. These include peripheral and central pain processing, systemic metabolic dysfunction and obesity, and aging-associated cellular senescence, all of which are increasingly implicated in OA pathophysiology and have informed distinct therapeutic strategies over the past decade.[9,10,13] We also review contemporary intra-articular regenerative approaches, including platelet-rich plasma (PRP), hyaluronic acid (HA), lubricin, and cell-based products, which are used in practice but require careful evaluation of their supporting evidence. Together, the 2 parts of the review are intended to provide a broad synthesis of current and emerging therapeutic targets for OA.

NERVE- AND NOCICEPTION-TARGETED THERAPIES

Nerve growth factor (NGF)–tropomyosin receptor kinase A (TrkA) signaling is a validated peripheral pain pathway. Tanezumab is a humanized monoclonal antibody that sequesters NGF, thereby reducing NGF–TrkA–mediated peripheral nociceptor sensitization and downstream pain amplification in hip and knee OA. In a large phase 3 trial in hip/knee OA, subcutaneous tanezumab improved pain and function, but was accompanied by a higher frequency of adjudicated rapidly progressive OA, reinforcing a narrow therapeutic window. This risk–benefit tension shaped the regulatory outcome: a U.S. Food and Drug Administration (FDA) advisory committee voted against approval in 2021.[14–16] Parallel programs with fasinumab have similarly demonstrated statistically significant improvements in WOMAC pain and physical function in knee/hip OA, while continuing to highlight adverse arthropathies and joint safety events that appear dose-related and require vigilant imaging-based eligibility/surveillance.[17,18] Collectively, anti-NGF therapies provide strong proof-of-mechanism for peripheral pain biology but remain constrained by joint safety liabilities that complicate broad adoption.

Beyond anti-NGF antibodies, nociceptive targeting in OA has advanced through local peripheral defunctionalization and neuromodulation approaches. Intra-articular transcapsaicin (CNTX-4975; Transient receptor potential cation channel subfamily V member 1 (TRPV1) agonism) produced dose-dependent improvements in knee OA pain, with the 1.0 mg dose showing benefit through 24 weeks in a randomized, placebo-controlled trial.[19] Central pain modulation remains clinically relevant, with randomized trials showing that duloxetine can reduce chronic knee and hip OA pain and improve function, consistent with its role in addressing centralized pain amplification in selected patients.[20] For procedural denervation, genicular nerve radiofrequency ablation has demonstrated symptomatic and functional improvements in sham-controlled randomized trials in knee OA with a favorable safety profile.[21]

SYSTEMIC METABOLIC TARGETS

Obesity contributes to knee and hip OA through combined biomechanical loading and systemic metabolic inflammation (insulin resistance, adipokine signaling, low-grade cytokine tone) that can amplify synovitis, osteochondral remodeling, and pain sensitivity, supporting a clinically actionable *metabolic OA* phenotype. Lifestyle programs remain foundational: in IDEA randomized controlled trial (RCT), intensive diet-induced weight loss, with or without exercise, improved symptoms and reduced knee joint loading in overweight and obese adults with knee OA.[22] The STEP 9 trial provides high-quality evidence that systemic metabolic modification can yield clinically relevant OA outcomes. The strongest pharmacologic signal to date is STEP 9 RCT, where once-weekly semaglutide 2.4 mg in adults with obesity and symptomatic knee OA produced substantially greater weight loss and WOMAC pain improvement than placebo at 68 weeks.[23] A 2025 randomized clinical trial found that metformin 2000 mg/day reduced knee pain more than placebo at 6 months in overweight/obese patients with symptomatic knee OA.[24] Ongoing trials are now designed to test whether potent antiobesity agents can affect hard outcomes like progression to arthroplasty, exemplified by a large tirzepatide trial (NCT06191848) with a primary endpoint of knee replacement at 72 weeks.

SENESCENCE-TARGETED THERAPIES

Aging increases OA risk via multiple converging mechanisms: accumulated matrix damage, mitochondrial dysfunction, impaired autophagy, and expansion of senescent cells that produce a proinflammatory senescence-associated secretory phenotype (SASP).[25] SASP factors can amplify synovial inflammation, drive catabolic programs in cartilage, alter subchondral remodeling, and sensitize nociceptors, making senescence an attractive whole-joint, mechanism-based target that conceptually aligns with OA as a chronic, heterogeneous disease.

Senolytics (UBX0101), an intra-articular senolytic strategy targeting the MDM2–p53 interaction, showed acceptable tolerability and dose-associated improvements in pain/function in early human testing,[26] but UNITY reported that a larger randomized phase 2 knee OA study did not meet its 12-week WOMAC pain endpoint, and the program did not advance.[27] More recently, a phase I/II randomized trial (NCT04210986) of intermittent oral fisetin (a repurposed senolytic) in knee OA, found no benefit for pain, function, or MRI cartilage outcomes over 12 months despite a reassuring safety profile, underscoring the need for demonstrable target engagement, better joint delivery, and phenotype enrichment before senescence-directed therapy can be credibly positioned for hip or knee OA.

OTHER INTRA-ARTICULAR REGENERATIVE THERAPIES

Platelet-Rich Plasma

PRP is an autologous intra-articular orthobiologic intended to modulate the osteoarthritic joint environment by delivering concentrated platelet-derived growth factors and mediators that may dampen low-grade inflammation and support tissue repair.[28–30] In knee OA, meta-analyses of randomized trials generally report modest-to-moderate improvements in pain and function versus HA or corticosteroid injections through ~6 to 12 months, but with very high heterogeneity driven by inconsistent PRP preparation and injection protocols.[31,32] The blinded RESTORE placebo-controlled RCT found that an intra-articular PRP series did not improve pain or medial tibial cartilage volume at 12 months versus saline, reinforcing that efficacy is not uniform and may depend on phenotype/severity and trial design.[33] In hip OA, the evidence base is smaller; pooled RCT data have not shown clear superiority of PRP over HA for pain or function.[34] Across studies, adverse events are typically limited to transient postinjection pain/swelling; leukocyte-rich preparations may be associated with more local reactions.[32] Clinically, PRP is best positioned as a symptom-modifying intra-articular option rather than a definitive disease-modifying therapy. Its use is most defensible in selected patients, particularly those with milder disease, while the field continues to address key limitations. Practical adoption also depends on value: current pricing and marketing often outpace the strength and consistency of clinical data, and cost-effectiveness remains uncertain, largely because it is not yet clear whether PRP meaningfully delays progression to arthroplasty.[30]

Intra-articular Hyaluronan/Hyaluronic Acid

The rationale for intra-articular HA is as a viscosupplement and biologic lubricant with proposed anti-inflammatory and analgesic effects, and it remains a symptom-modifying option rather than a proven disease modifier.[35,36] In knee OA, systematic reviews show that repeated courses can maintain or further improve pain relief without an increased safety signal over time.[37] However, the average benefit is modest: compared with oral nonsteroidal anti-inflammatory drugs (NSAIDs), HA provides statistically significant but generally not clinically important improvements in pain and function, while offering a lower overall adverse-event risk.[38] Some analyses suggest higher–molecular weight HA achieves larger symptomatic effects than lower–molecular weight products, though findings are not uniform across studies.[39] For hip OA, the evidence base is smaller and more variable; recent syntheses of RCTs do not consistently demonstrate clear superiority of HA over comparators, supporting a more selective role when used.[40]

An additional approach evaluated preclinically that also seeks to improve joint tribology (frictional property) in OA is injection of recombinant lubricin or proteoglycan 4 (PRG4), a major contributor to low-friction in the joint, as well as to cartilage integrity and health.[41] Injection of lubricin into animal models of post-traumatic OA demonstrated a chondroprotective effect in rats[42,43] and Yucatan minipigs[44] and in a rabbit model of temporomandibular joint OA.[45] However, there appear to be no active clinical trials on the use of lubricin as a therapeutic in OA.

Cell-Based Therapies

Cell–based therapies for OA span minimally manipulated autologous products (e.g., bone marrow aspirate concentrate/bone marrow–derived cell preparations and adipose stromal vascular fraction) as well as culture-expanded mesenchymal stem cells (MSCs), which differ substantially in composition, processing, dosing, and oversight.[46] In knee OA, multiple meta-analyses (including RCT-focused reviews) generally show short-term improvements in pain and patient-reported function (Visual Analog Scale [VAS], Western Ontario and McMaster Universities Osteoarthritis Index [WOMAC]/ Knee injury and Osteoarthritis Outcome Score [KOOS]), but structural outcomes are inconsistent; cartilage volume may increase in some analyses while compositional MRI scores often do not, highlighting heterogeneity and limited high-quality evidence for true disease modification.[47–49] In hip OA, the clinical evidence base is much smaller, with signals for symptomatic benefit but insufficient evidence for durable structure modification.[50,51] While early clinical studies indicate that intra-articular cellular injections are generally safe with no major adverse events and can provide modest improvements in pain and function, the current evidence remains largely at the proof-of-concept stage.[52,53] The existing literature is significantly limited by poor methodological quality, a lack of standardized cell characterization, high heterogeneity in cell processing techniques, and the inability to completely rule out a strong placebo effect. Furthermore, despite misleading marketing claims from commercial clinics promising "cartilage regeneration", the primary mechanism of action is increasingly believed to rely on paracrine and immunomodulatory effects, wherein secreted cytokines and growth factors alter the intra-articular milieu to reduce inflammation, rather than true stem cell engraftment and new tissue formation.[54]

Clinically, patients should be counseled that efficacy and durability remain uncertain, that online or direct-to-consumer information can overstate benefits and omit key risks or cost considerations, and that professional society positions caution against routine use for advanced hip or knee arthritis outside well-designed trials/registries.[55–57]

DRUG DELIVERY

A central reason why many OA candidates fail is not target selection alone, it is drug delivery and target engagement. The joint clears soluble injectables rapidly via synovial capillaries and lymphatics, and many molecules do not penetrate cartilage effectively. Extended-release intra-articular corticosteroid microspheres (FX006/ TA-ER) demonstrate the principle that modifying residence time can extend symptom benefit compared with saline at clinically relevant timepoints.[58] Looking ahead, scalable platforms like hydrogels, nanoparticles, and depot formulations should be evaluated as enabling technologies for both anti-inflammatory and structure-directed agents.[59] Local gene-based expression represents a transformative delivery solution in disguise. For instance, intra-articular sc-rAAV2.5 IL-1 receptor antagonist has demonstrated the potential for sustained, endogenous therapeutic expression with a reassuring Phase 1 safety profile.[60]

EXPERT OPINION

The current state of OA research is at a critical inflection point. While the review correctly identifies several biologically compelling targets, the translational *valley of death*, where promising Phase 2 signals fail to achieve Phase 3 success, remains our greatest hurdle. Overcoming this challenge will require a fundamental shift in how OA is defined, studied, and treated. In particular a weakness of most current therapy trials is the assumption that a drug of intervention will work equally well for all patients, because it assumes that the underlying mechanisms in ongoing OA in each individual are the same. Further progress will therefore require tighter integration of clinical phenotyping with biomarker- and omics-based approaches to define narrower patient categories for clinical trials. However, direct evidence for reproducible molecular endotypes in knee OA remains limited, and further investigation in well-defined cohorts with distinct clinical phenotypes is warranted before endotype-guided therapeutic stratification can be realized.[12,61] As one example, the proteolytic landscape of osteoarthritic cartilage is highly complex. Emerging omics technologies are now beginning to characterize this process with greater molecular precision. Forward and reverse degradomics, for instance, can identify extensive protease-specific cleavage patterns across cartilage and synovial fluid, providing insight into the relative contributions of enzymes such as

HtrA1, ADAMTS5, MMP13, and CMA1.[62,63] These proteases are only among a handful of numerous proteases that may contribute to stage/patient/joint specific patterns of cartilage breakdown and inflammation. A better grasp of proteolytic biomarkers may help to refine patient-specific, mechanism-based therapeutic targeting, rather a *one-drug fits all* concept, where drugs with relatively small but still beneficial effects, may be predestined to failure.

By integrating high-dimensional omics data with clinical metrics, imaging, and patient-reported outcome measures, it may become possible to develop digital twins for OA.[64] These patient-specific computational models could mirror the biological and clinical state of an individual patient, allowing investigators to model disease progression and evaluate targeted interventions in silico before they are used in practice. Ultimately, we must stop asking "Does this drug work for OA?" and start asking "Which patients, defined by their clinical presentation and supported by mechanism-relevant biomarkers, are most likely to benefit?"

The human cost of OA and its end-stage complications, such as periprosthetic infections or persistent post-surgical pain, is staggering. This burden will only grow as populations age and the prevalence of OA rises. In that context, arthroplasty and the broader care of advanced OA should no longer be viewed narrowly as elective or isolated orthopedic concerns, but as part of a larger public health and health-systems challenge.[65] To combat this, we need multidisciplinary Centers of Excellence that unite orthopedic surgeons, biologists, data scientists, and other subspecialties. We must also advocate for research funding that matches the massive economic and social burden of musculoskeletal disease, which currently receives less than 2% of NIH funds despite affecting one-third of the population.[66,67] The future of OA management lies at the intersection of precision personalized medicine and patient-centric care.[68] By using data to optimize patient selection and setting expectations through predictive modeling, we can ensure that the innovative therapies described in this review finally reach the patients who need them most.

SUMMARY

This review highlights osteoarthritis (OA) as a heterogeneous whole-joint disease shaped by pain pathways, metabolic dysfunction, cellular senescence, and regenerative intra-articular treatment approaches. While several emerging therapies show mechanistic promise, durable clinical benefit remains limited, emphasizing the need for better patient stratification, biomarker-guided trials, and improved drug-delivery systems to support more precise OA care.

CLINICS CARE POINTS

- Osteoarthritis (OA) should be managed as a whole-patient condition, with attention to systemic and extra-articular contributors such as obesity, metabolic dysfunction, pain sensitization, and aging biology.
- Regenerative and orthobiologic therapies should be positioned carefully: Patients should be counseled that evidence remains heterogeneous, durability is uncertain, and commercial claims may exceed the strength of available data.
- Drug delivery is a central therapeutic issue in OA: Failure of an OA therapy may reflect inadequate joint residence time or poor tissue penetration. Sustained-release intra-articular platforms, biomaterial-based depots, and local gene-based expression systems may prove critical to improving target engagement and translating promising mechanisms into clinically meaningful benefit.
- Pitfall: The promise of precision medicine in OA is substantial, but its implementation should not outpace the evidence. While clinical phenotyping already offers a useful framework for patient stratification, the field is still working to determine whether reproducible molecular endotypes can be robustly defined and meaningfully linked to treatment response. Clearly, even the last word on molecular endotyping has not been written given the many advances still needed for truly understanding the molecular biology of OA.

DISCLOSURE

N.S. Piuzzi has the following disclosures not related to the present study: Grants or contracts – Osteal Therapeutics, Peptilogics, RegenLab, Signature Orthopedics, Zimmer, United States, and Stryker, United States; Consulting fees – Zimmer, Pacira Pharmaceutical, and Stryker; Editorial board member or Leadership role – *JBJS, American Association of Hip and Knee Surgeons, and Orthopaedic Research Society*. All the other authors have no disclosures.

REFERENCES

1. Lespasio MJ, Sultan AA, Piuzzi NS, et al. Hip osteoarthritis: a primer. Perm J 2018;22(1):17–084.

2. Lespasio MJ, Piuzzi NS, Husni ME, et al. Knee osteoarthritis: a primer. Perm J 2017;21:16–183. PubMed PMID: 29035179; PubMed Central PMCID: PMC5638628.
3. Dieleman JL, Baral R, Birger M, et al. US spending on personal health care and public health, 1996-2013. JAMA 2016;316(24):2627–46. PubMed PMID: 28027366; PubMed Central PMCID: PMC5551483.
4. GBD 2021 Osteoarthritis Collaborators. Global, regional, and national burden of osteoarthritis, 1990-2020 and projections to 2050: a systematic analysis for the global burden of disease study 2021. Lancet Rheumatol 2023;5(9):e508–22.
5. Loeser RF, Goldring SR, Scanzello CR, et al. Osteoarthritis: a disease of the joint as an organ. Arthritis Rheum 2012;64(6):1697–707. PubMed PMID: 2239 2533; PubMed Central PMCID: PMC3366018.
6. Hunter DJ, Bierma-Zeinstra S. Osteoarthritis. Lancet 2019;393(10182):1745–59.
7. Cho Y, Jeong S, Kim H, et al. Disease-modifying therapeutic strategies in osteoarthritis: current status and future directions. Exp Mol Med 2021;53(11): 1689–96. PubMed PMID: 34848838; PubMed Central PMCID: PMC8640059.
8. Kolasinski SL, Neogi T, Hochberg MC, et al. 2019 American college of rheumatology/Arthritis Foundation Guideline for the management of osteoarthritis of the hand, hip, and knee. Arthritis Care Res 2020;72(2):149–62. PubMed PMID: 31908149; PubMed Central PMCID: PMC11488261.
9. Van Spil WE, Kubassova O, Boesen M, et al. Osteoarthritis phenotypes and novel therapeutic targets. Biochem Pharmacol 2019;165:41–8.
10. Brandt MD, Malone JB, Kean TJ. Advances and challenges in the pursuit of disease-modifying osteoarthritis drugs: a review of 2010–2024 clinical trials. Biomedicines 2025;13(2). https://doi.org/10.3390/biomedicines13020355.
11. Mobasheri A, Loeser R. Clinical phenotypes, molecular endotypes and theratypes in OA therapeutic development. Nat Rev Rheumatol 2024;20(9): 525–6.
12. Perry TA, Deng Y, Hulley P, et al. Deconvoluting synovial fluid molecular endotypes in knee osteoarthritis: primary results from the STEpUP OA consortium. medRxiv 2024. https://doi.org/10.1101/2024.06.05.24308485 [cited 2026 Mar 24]. p. 2024.06.05.2430 8485. Available at: https://www.medrxiv.org/content/10.1101/2024.06.05.24308485v2.
13. Mantripragada VP, Csorba A, Bova W, et al. Assessment of clinical, tissue, and cell-level metrics identify four biologically distinct knee osteoarthritis patient phenotypes. Cartilage 2022;13(1):1947603 5221074003. PubMed PMID: 35109693; PubMed Central PMCID: PMC9137310.
14. Taylor NP. Lilly, Pfizer stop development of osteoarthritis drug after FDA rejection, extending bleak run for NGF inhibitors. Fierce Biotech; 2021 [cited 2026 Jan 29]. Available at: https://www.fiercebiotech.com/biotech/lilly-pfizer-stop-development-osteoarthritis-drug-after-fda-rejection-extending-bleak-run.
15. Berenbaum F, Blanco FJ, Guermazi A, et al. Subcutaneous tanezumab for osteoarthritis of the hip or knee: efficacy and safety results from a 24-week randomised phase III study with a 24-week follow-up period. Ann Rheum Dis 2020;79(6):800–10.
16. Roemer FW, Hochberg MC, Carrino JA, et al. Role of imaging for eligibility and safety of a-NGF clinical trials. Ther Adv Musculoskelet Dis 2023;15: 1759720X231171768. PubMed PMID: 37284331; PubMed Central PMCID: PMC10240557.
17. Dakin P, DiMartino SJ, Gao H, et al. The efficacy, tolerability, and joint safety of fasinumab in osteoarthritis pain: a phase IIb/III double-blind, placebo-controlled, randomized clinical trial. Arthritis Rheumatol 2019;71-(11):1824–34.
18. DiMartino SJ, Mei J, Schnitzer TJ, et al. A phase III study to evaluate the long-term safety and efficacy of fasinumab in patients with pain due to osteoarthritis of the knee or hip. Osteoarthr Cartil Open 2024;6(4):100533. PubMed PMID: 39554479; PubMed Central PMCID: PMC11566341.
19. Stevens RM, Ervin J, Nezzer J, et al. Randomized, double blind, placebo controlled trial of intraarticular trans capsaicin for pain associated with osteoarthritis of the knee. Arthritis Rheumatol Hoboken Nj 2019;71(9):1524–33. PubMed PMID: 30888737; PubMed Central PMCID: PMC 6772016.
20. Chappell AS, Desaiah D, Liu-Seifert H, et al. A double-blind, randomized, placebo-controlled study of the efficacy and safety of duloxetine for the treatment of chronic pain due to osteoarthritis of the knee. Pain Pract 2011;11(1):33–41.
21. Barreto RB, Barreto A de J, do Nascimento ALM, et al. Efficacy and safety of genicular nerve ablation techniques for knee osteoarthritis: a systematic review and meta-analysis of Sham-controlled randomized trials. Pain Med 2026;27(4):449–61.
22. Messier SP, Mihalko SL, Legault C, et al. Effects of intensive diet and exercise on knee joint loads, inflammation, and clinical outcomes among overweight and Obese adults with knee osteoarthritis: the IDEA randomized clinical trial. JAMA 2013;310-(12):1263–73.
23. Bliddal H, Bays H, Czernichow S, et al, STEP 9 Study Group. Once-weekly semaglutide in persons with obesity and knee osteoarthritis. N Engl J Med 2024;391(17):1573–83.
24. Pan F, Wang Y, Lim YZ, et al. Metformin for knee osteoarthritis in patients with overweight or obesity: a randomized clinical trial. JAMA 2025;333-(20):1804–12.

25. Cai X, Yuan S, Zeng Y, et al. New trends in pharmacological treatments for osteoarthritis. Front Pharmacol 2021;12. https://doi.org/10.3389/fphar.2021.645842.
26. Safety, tolerability, pharmacokinetics, and clinical outcomes following single-dose IA administration of UBX0101, a senolytic MDM2/p53 interaction inhibitor, in patients with knee OA. ACR meeting abstracts [Internet] [cited 2026 Jan 29]. Available at: https://acrabstracts.org/abstract/safety-tolerability-pharmacokinetics-and-clinical-outcomes-following-single-dose-ia-administration-of-ubx0101-a-senolytic-mdm2-p53-interaction-inhibitor-in-patients-with-knee-oa/.
27. Inc UB. GlobeNewswire News Room [Internet]. UNITY biotechnology announces 12-week data from UBX0101 phase 2 clinical study in patients with painful osteoarthritis of the knee. 2020 [cited 2026 Jan 29]. Available at: https://www.globenewswire.com/news-release/2020/08/17/2079116/0/en/UNITY-Biotechnology-Announces-12-week-data-from-UBX0101-Phase-2-Clinical-Study-in-Patients-with-Painful-Osteoarthritis-of-the-Knee.html.
28. Oliveira L, King D, Genin J, et al. What is the efficacy of intra-articular platelet-rich plasma injections for knee osteoarthritis in clinical practice? A "Real-Life" prospective cohort. Surg Technol Int 2023;43:267–71.
29. Leal C, Chahla J, Rossi L, et al. From platelet-rich plasma to mesenchymal stem cells: cartilage, tendon, and bone regeneration with orthobiologics. Instr Course Lect 2024;73:3–13.
30. Rajan PV, Ng MK, Klika A, et al. The cost-effectiveness of platelet-rich plasma injections for knee osteoarthritis: a markov decision analysis. J Bone Joint Surg Am 2020;102(18):e104. PubMed PMID: 32453118.
31. Khalid S, Ali A, Deepak F, et al. Comparative effectiveness of intra-articular therapies in knee osteoarthritis: a meta-analysis comparing platelet-rich plasma (PRP) with other treatment modalities. Ann Med Surg 2023;86(1):361–72. PubMed PMID: 38222750; PubMed Central PMCID: PMC10783230.
32. Kim JH, Park YB, Ha CW. Are leukocyte-poor or multiple injections of platelet-rich plasma more effective than hyaluronic acid for knee osteoarthritis? A systematic review and meta-analysis of randomized controlled trials. Arch Orthop Trauma Surg 2023;143(7):3879–97.
33. Bennell KL, Paterson KL, Metcalf BR, et al. Effect of intra-articular platelet-rich plasma vs placebo injection on pain and medial tibial cartilage volume in patients with knee osteoarthritis. JAMA 2021;326(20):1–11. PubMed PMID: 34812863; PubMed Central PMCID: PMC8611484.
34. Belk JW, Houck DA, Littlefield CP, et al. Platelet-rich plasma versus hyaluronic acid for hip osteoarthritis yields similarly beneficial short-term clinical outcomes: a systematic review and meta-analysis of level I and II randomized controlled trials. Arthrosc J Arthrosc Relat Surg 2022;38(6):2035–46.
35. Shtroblia V, Petakh P, Kamyshna I, et al. Recent advances in the management of knee osteoarthritis: a narrative review. Front Med 2025;12. https://doi.org/10.3389/fmed.2025.1523027.
36. Piuzzi NS, Midura RJ, Muschler GF, et al. Intra-articular hyaluronan injections for the treatment of osteoarthritis: perspective for the mechanism of action. Ther Adv Musculoskelet Dis 2018;10(2):55–7.
37. Altman R, Hackel J, Niazi F, et al. Efficacy and safety of repeated courses of hyaluronic acid injections for knee osteoarthritis: a systematic review. Semin Arthritis Rheum 2018;48(2):168–75.
38. Miller LE, Fredericson M, Altman RD. Hyaluronic acid injections or oral nonsteroidal anti-inflammatory drugs for knee osteoarthritis: systematic review and meta-analysis of randomized trials. Orthop J Sports Med 2020;8(1):2325967119897909. PubMed PMID: 32047830; PubMed Central PMCID: PMC6985976.
39. Hummer C, Angst F, Schemitsch E, et al. High molecular weight intraarticular hyaluronic acid for the treatment of knee osteoarthritis: network meta-analysis. Osteoarthr Cartil 2019;27:S503–4.
40. Migliorini F, Pilone M, Mazzoleni MG, et al. Intra-articular hyaluronic acid injections for hip osteoarthritis: a level I systematic review. Eur J Orthop Surg Traumatol 2025;35(1):180. PubMed PMID: 40343507; PubMed Central PMCID: PMC12064613.
41. Jay GD, Waller KA. The biology of lubricin: near frictionless joint motion. Matrix Biol J Int Soc Matrix Biol 2014;39:17–24.
42. Jay GD, Fleming BC, Watkins BA, et al. Prevention of cartilage degeneration and restoration of chondroprotection by lubricin tribosupplementation in the rat following anterior cruciate ligament transection. Arthritis Rheum 2010;62(8):2382–91. PubMed PMID: 20506144; PubMed Central PMCID: PMC2921027.
43. Elsaid KA, Zhang L, Shaman Z, et al. The impact of early intra-articular administration of interleukin-1 receptor antagonist on lubricin metabolism and cartilage degeneration in an anterior cruciate ligament transection model. Osteoarthr Cartil 2015;23(1):114–21. PubMed PMID: 25219670; PubMed Central PMCID: PMC4275352.
44. Waller KA, Chin KE, Jay GD, et al. Intra-articular recombinant human proteoglycan 4 mitigates cartilage damage after destabilization of the medial meniscus in the Yucatan minipig. Am J Sports Med 2017;45(7):1512–21. PubMed PMID: 28129516; PubMed Central PMCID: PMC5453820.
45. Iturriaga V, Vásquez B, Wen S, et al. Intra-articular administration of recombinant human proteoglycan

4 (rhPRG4) as a potential therapy for temporomandibular joint osteoarthritis: a preclinical histopathological study. Int J Mol Sci 2025;26(19):9305. PubMed PMID: 41096574; PubMed Central PMCID: PMC12524758.
46. Piuzzi NS, Ng M, Chughtai M, et al. Accelerated growth of cellular therapy trials in musculoskeletal disorders: an analysis of the NIH clinical trials data bank. Orthopedics 2019;42(2):e144–50.
47. Ma W, Liu C, Wang S, et al. Efficacy and safety of intra-articular injection of mesenchymal stem cells in the treatment of knee osteoarthritis: a systematic review and meta-analysis. Medicine (Baltim) 2020; 99(49):e23343.
48. Kim SH, Djaja YP, Park YB, et al. Intra-articular injection of culture-expanded mesenchymal stem cells without adjuvant surgery in knee osteoarthritis: a systematic review and meta-analysis. Am J Sports Med 2020;48(11):2839–49.
49. Kim SH, Ha CW, Park YB, et al. Intra-articular injection of mesenchymal stem cells for clinical outcomes and cartilage repair in osteoarthritis of the knee: a meta-analysis of randomized controlled trials. Arch Orthop Trauma Surg 2019; 139(7):971–80.
50. Giorgino R, Alessandri Bonetti M, Migliorini F, et al. Management of hip osteoarthritis: harnessing the potential of mesenchymal stem cells-a systematic review. Eur J Orthop Surg Traumatol Orthop Traumatol 2024;34(8):3847–57. PubMed PMID: 39254726; PubMed Central PMCID: PMC 11519189.
51. Entessari M, Oliveira LP. Current evidence on mesenchymal stem cells for hip osteoarthritis: a narrative review. Regen Med 2023;18(9):749–58.
52. Chahla J, Piuzzi NS, Mitchell JJ, et al. Intra-articular cellular therapy for osteoarthritis and focal cartilage defects of the knee: a systematic review of the literature and study quality analysis. J Bone Joint Surg Am 2016;98(18):1511–21.
53. Piuzzi NS, Khlopas A, Newman JM, et al. Bone marrow cellular therapies: novel therapy for knee osteoarthritis. J Knee Surg 2018;31(1):22–6.
54. Murray IR, Chahla J, Frank RM, et al. Rogue stem cell clinics. Bone Jt J 2020;102-B(2):148–54. PubMed PMID: 32009438; PubMed Central PMCID: PMC70 02842.
55. Chu CR, Rodeo S, Bhutani N, et al. Optimizing clinical use of biologics in orthopaedic surgery: consensus recommendations from the 2018 AAOS/NIH U-13 conference. J Am Acad Orthop Surg 2019;27(2): e50–63. PubMed PMID: 30300216; PubMed Central PMCID: PMC6314629.
56. Piuzzi NS, Emara A, Chahla J, et al. Ethical and practical considerations for integrating cellular ("stem cell") therapy into clinical practice. Curr Rev Musculoskelet Med 2020;13(4):525–9. PubMed PMID: 32468421; PubMed Central PMCID: PMC 7340700.
57. Ng MK, Mont MA, Piuzzi NS. Analysis of readability, quality, and content of online information available for "Stem Cell" injections for knee osteoarthritis. J Arthroplast 2020;35(3):647–51.e2.
58. Conaghan PG, Hunter DJ, Cohen SB, et al. Effects of a single intra-articular injection of a microsphere formulation of triamcinolone acetonide on knee osteoarthritis pain. J Bone Joint Surg Am 2018; 100(8):666–77. PubMed PMID: 29664853; PubMed Central PMCID: PMC5916484.
59. Huang H, Lou Z, Zheng S, et al. Intra-articular drug delivery systems for osteoarthritis therapy: shifting from sustained release to enhancing penetration into cartilage. Drug Deliv 2022;29(1):767–91. PubMed PMID: 35261301; PubMed Central PMCID: PMC8920370.
60. De la Vega RE, Sellon JL, Smith J, et al. A phase 1 clinical trial shows safe, sustained, AAV-mediated expression of IL-1Ra in the human osteoarthritic knee joint. Sci Transl Med 2025;17(801): eadu9804.
61. Steinberg J, Southam L, Fontalis A, et al. Linking chondrocyte and synovial transcriptional profile to clinical phenotype in osteoarthritis. Ann Rheum Dis 2021;80(8):1070–4. PubMed PMID: 33903094; PubMed Central PMCID: PMC8292595.
62. Bhutada S, Hoyle A, Piuzzi NS, et al. Degradomics defines proteolysis information flow from human knee osteoarthritis cartilage to matched synovial fluid and the contributions of secreted proteases ADAMTS5, MMP13 and CMA1 to articular cartilage breakdown. Osteoarthr Cartil 2025;33(1):116–27. PubMed PMID: 39293776; PubMed Central PMCID: PMC12342059.
63. Bhutada S, Li L, Willard B, et al. Forward and reverse degradomics defines the proteolytic landscape of human knee osteoarthritic cartilage and the role of the serine protease HtrA1. Osteoarthr Cartil 2022;30(8):1091–102.
64. Jayakumar P, Rathouz PJ, Lin E, et al. Shared decision making using digital twins in knee osteoarthritis care: a randomized clinical trial of an AI-enabled decision aid versus education alone on decision quality, physical function, and user experience. eClinicalMedicine 2025;89:103545. PubMed PMID: 41112505; PubMed Central PMCID: PMC12528923.
65. Delaney PG, Piuzzi NS. A call for inclusion of arthroplasty as essential surgery. Bull World Health Organ 2026;104(4):274–81. PubMed PMID: 41924341; PubMed Central PMCID: PMC13037251.
66. Ng MK, Rullan-Oliver P, Magruder M, et al. Comparison of industry and national institutes of health funding for orthopedic surgery research. Orthopedics 2025;48(4):e182–6.

67. McConaghy K, Klika AK, Apte SS, et al. A call to action for musculoskeletal research funding: the growing economic and disease burden of musculoskeletal conditions in the United States is not reflected in musculoskeletal research funding. J Bone Joint Surg Am 2023;105(6):492–8.

68. Khan ST, Huffman N, Li X, et al. Pain assessment in osteoarthritis: present practices and future prospects including the use of biomarkers and wearable technologies, and AI-Driven personalized medicine. J Orthop Res 2025;43(7):1217–29. PubMed PMID: 40205648; PubMed Central PMCID: PMC12159590.

The Role of Platelet-rich Plasma in the Treatment of Osteoarthritis of the Knee

Warran Wignadasan, MBBS, FRCS(Orth),
Taewoong Chae, MD,
Michael E. Neufeld, MD, FRCSC, MSc,
Lisa C. Howard, MD, MHSc, FRCSC,
Bassam A. Masri, MD, FRCSC*

KEYWORDS

• Platelet-rich plasma (PRP) • Hyaluronic acid • NF-κB • Osteoarthritis • Knee osteoarthritis

KEY POINTS

- Platelet-rich plasma (PRP) is a biologically plausible therapy with anti-inflammatory and analgesic effects, but clinical outcomes are heterogeneous.
- Disease-modifying effects remain unproven, with conflicting imaging evidence.
- PRP is best considered in selected patients seeking to delay surgery, rather than as routine therapy.

INTRODUCTION

Knee osteoarthritis (OA) is a prevalent, progressive musculoskeletal disorder and a leading cause of pain, disability, and reduced quality of life worldwide.[1] With an aging population, coupled with rising rates of obesity, the global burden of knee OA continues to increase, placing significant strain on health care systems.[2] From a pathophysiological standpoint, knee OA is no longer regarded as a purely degenerative condition, but rather a complex disease process involving cartilage degradation, synovial inflammation, subchondral bone remodeling and altered joint biomechanics.[3] Despite advances in understanding disease mechanisms, current treatment strategies remain largely focused on symptom control rather than disease modification.

Nonoperative management options for knee OA include lifestyle modification, physical therapy, analgesics and intra-articular injections. Corticosteroids and hyaluronic acid (HA) are widely utilized injectable therapies; however, their clinical benefits are often short-lived and variable with persisting concerns regarding potential effects with repeated use.[4,5] Although knee arthroplasty remains the gold standard treatment of end-stage knee OA, there is growing patient interest in nonoperative measures, including injections. This shift reflects a desire to delay or avoid surgery due to concerns regarding surgical risk, recovery time, implant longevity, costs, as well as the increasing prevalence of younger, more active patients with symptomatic disease.

Platelet-rich plasma (PRP) has emerged as an orthobiologic treatment of knee OA.[6] Derived from autologous blood, PRP contains a concentrated suspension of platelets and bioactive molecules, including growth factors and cytokines, which may exert anti-inflammatory and anabolic effects within the osteoarthritic joint.[7] Preclinical studies suggest that PRP may

Department of Orthopaedics, University of British Columbia, M430-2211 Wesbrook Mall, Vancouver, BC V6T 2B5, Canada
* Corresponding author.
E-mail address: bas.masri@vch.ca

Orthop Clin N Am 57 (2026) 299–306
https://doi.org/10.1016/j.ocl.2026.05.005

Abbreviations	
BMI	body mass index
HA	hyaluronic acid
IL-1 β	interleukin-1 beta
LP-PRP	leukocyte-poor PRP
LR-PRP	leukocyte-rich PRP
NF-κB	nuclear factor kappa light chain enhancer of activated B cells
OA	osteoarthritis
PRP	platelet-rich plasma
RCTs	randomized controlled trials
TNF-α	tumor necrosis factor-alpha
WBCs	white blood cells
WOMAC	Western Ontario and McMaster Universities Osteoarthritis Index

modulate synovial inflammation, influence chondrocyte metabolism and support cartilage homeostasis.[8,9] Over the last decade, an increasing number of clinical studies have investigated the efficacy of PRP injections in knee OA, with variability in the results reported.[10–13]

The aim of this review is to synthesize the current biological rationale and clinical evidence supporting the use of PRP in the management of knee OA, critically appraise existing limitations, and discuss its evolving role in contemporary clinical practice.

BIOLOGICAL BASIS OF PLATELET-RICH PLASMA

PRP is an autologous blood product containing a platelet concentration several-fold above baseline levels.[14] While significant variability exists among commercial PRP formulations regarding collection and preparation, the core mechanism remains consistent: upon activation, platelets degranulate, releasing an array of bioactive molecules, including growth factors, cytokines, and chemokines.[14] These factors modulate inflammation in chondrocytes and synoviocytes, cartilage metabolism, and nociception.[14,15]

PRP's anti-inflammatory effects largely target the nuclear factor kappa light chain enhancer of activated B cells (NF-κB) pathway. This group of transcription factors is implicated in the inflammatory and catabolic processes of OA.[16] The NF-κB pathway integrates mechanical stress and proinflammatory signals, driving the expression of matrix metalloproteinases, cytokines, and proapoptotic genes that promote cartilage destruction and synovitis.[16] In osteoarthritic chondrocytes, proinflammatory cytokines such as tumor necrosis factor-alpha (TNF-α) and interleukin-1 beta (IL-1 β) activate the NF-κB pathway, accelerating extracellular matrix degradation and chondrocyte catabolism.[16] Within synoviocytes, this activation leads to synovitis, characterized by immune cell infiltration, further contributing to osteoarthritic pain.[16]

PRP modulates the NF-κB signaling pathway through both anti-inflammatory and proinflammatory components. IL-1 receptor antagonist inhibits IL-1β binding, reducing downstream inflammatory gene expression,[17] while hepatocyte growth factor further suppresses NF-κB activity in human chondrocytes.[18] However, PRP also contains proinflammatory mediators that may promote cartilage damage, synovitis, and osteophyte formation, reflecting its dualistic mechanism of action.[14] It also appears to modulate pain directly by targeting macrophages, which are implicated in synovitis and OA pain. Xu and colleagues[15] reported that PRP inhibits NF-κB activation in synovial macrophages and induces a phenotypic conversion from M1 (proinflammatory) to M2 (anti-inflammatory). M1 macrophages produce cytokines such as TNF-α and IL-1 β, whereas the M2 phenotype releases interleukin-10, an anti-inflammatory cytokine with analgesic properties.[15] Thus, PRP may contribute to the modulation of OA-related pain through an antinociceptive mechanism driven by macrophage polarization.

PRP exerts potentially disease-modifying effects by delivering a concentrated mix of anabolic growth factors—including platelet-derived growth factor, transforming growth factor-beta, and vascular endothelial growth factor—that support cartilage cell survival and matrix repair.[14] These factors promote chondrocyte and mesenchymal stem cell proliferation, enhance stem-cell recruitment to site of injury, and reduce chondrocyte apoptosis.[14] At the matrix level, PRP enhances the synthesis of type II collagen and proteoglycans, the primary structural components of hyaline cartilage.[14] It needs to be stressed that this is potentially disease-modifying, not disease reversing as regenerative medicine advocates often claim.

THE PREPARATION AND CLASSIFICATION OF PLATELET-RICH PLASMA

Despite extensive heterogeneity in preparation methods, the fundamental principle involves centrifugation of autologous, whole blood to separate the plasma fraction and concentrate platelets.[14] Compositional variability arises from procedural factors including centrifugal force, spin duration, number of spins (single vs double), and the final plasma volume collected.[19] Whether prepared by manual laboratory techniques or automated commercial systems, PRP products yield distinct cellular and biochemical profiles dependent on the technique, complicating the comparison of clinical outcomes across studies.[19]

To address this heterogeneity, multiple classification systems have been proposed. Ehrenfest and colleagues[20] introduced an early framework based on leukocyte content and fibrin architecture. Subsequent classification systems included the PAW classification (platelets, activation, white blood cells [WBCs]),[21] platelet to lymphocyte ratio (PLRA) classification (adding red blood cell concentration),[22] and DEPA (dose, efficiency, purity, activation).[23] More recently, the MARSPILL framework expanded criteria to include harvest technique, image guidance, and light activation.[24] Despite these efforts, no single framework has been universally adopted, underscoring the lack of standardization in the field.[25]

One of the most clinically relevant distinctions is leukocyte content. Leukocyte-poor PRP (LP-PRP) contains WBC levels at or below baseline, while leukocyte-rich PRP (LR-PRP) exceeds baseline levels.[21] Preclinical evidence initially suggested that LP-PRP was preferable for knee OA, as it appears to produce a less inflammatory environment.[26] Conversely, LR-PRP has been shown to increase synoviocyte death in vitro.[26]

Clinical evidence; however, remains inconsistent. While early data favored LP-PRP,[26] recent studies demonstrate no significant difference in efficacy between formulations.[27,28] Regarding safety, LR-PRP is associated with increased post-injection pain and swelling,[28] though recent studies found no significant difference in adverse event rates.[27] Consequently, the clinical superiority of one formulation over the other remains unresolved.

Platelet concentration is another critical variable. While preclinical models suggest higher concentrations enhance cartilage protection,[29] and some report improved outcomes with higher counts,[30] the relationship is likely nonlinear. PRP has been reported to have a plateau, and even inhibitory effect at supraphysiological concentrations, potentially disrupting cartilage homeostasis by overstimulating catabolic mediators.[31]

Activation, which triggers growth factor release, occurs exogenously (eg, calcium chloride and thrombin) or endogenously via exposure to joint collagen.[32] Exogenous activation causes rapid degranulation, whereas endogenous activation provides a sustained release.[32] Comparative studies are conflicting; some suggest collagen-mediated activation is superior,[21] while others favor calcium-based activators.[33] Clinically, evidence regarding the necessity of exogenous activation remains equivocal.[34]

CLINICAL EVIDENCE FOR PLATELET-RICH PLASMA IN KNEE OSTEOARTHRITIS

An expanding body of clinical literature has evaluated the efficacy of intra-articular PRP injections for the treatment of knee OA. Most available evidence consists of randomized controlled trials (RCTs) and prospective comparative studies, with outcome measures primarily focused on pain relief and functional improvement. Although heterogeneity in study design and PRP preparation remains a major limitation, the overall trend in the literature suggests that PRP may provide clinically meaningful symptomatic benefit, particularly in selected patient populations.

Symptomatic Outcomes

Multiple RCTs have demonstrated that PRP injections result in significant improvements in pain and function compared with baseline, as measured by validated outcome scores such as Visual Analogue Scale, Western Ontario and McMaster Universities Osteoarthritis Index (WOMAC) and Knee injury and Osteoarthritis Outcome Score.[10,35–38] Bensa and colleagues[30] conducted a meta-analysis of 18 RCTs and reported that PRP injections were associated with meaningful improvements in patient-reported outcome measures. The authors reported that a high-platelet PRP concentration was associated with prolonged benefits compared to low-platelet concentrations.

Platelet-rich Plasma Compared with Placebo and Saline

Several studies have evaluated intra-articular PRP against placebo or saline controls in patients with knee OA. Early studies reported significant improvements in pain and function following PRP injection compared with saline, as measured with validated outcome measures.[35] However, these findings have not been consistently replicated across subsequent trials, with considerable heterogeneity in study design, PRP preparation protocol, injection regimens and patient populations.[39] More recent, high-quality placebo-controlled studies have demonstrated limited to no meaningful differences between PRP and saline injections.[40] Collectively, these findings suggest that while PRP may provide short-term symptomatic improvement in some patients, its efficacy relative to placebo remains uncertain.

Platelet-rich Plasma versus Corticosteroid Injections

Corticosteroid injections are commonly used for short-term symptom control in patients with all levels of knee OA. Corticosteroid injections are consistently associated with rapid short-term improvements in pain and function, reflecting their potent anti-inflammatory effects; however, these benefits typically diminish within weeks to months.[41] In contrast, RCTs have suggested that PRP may provide more sustained symptomatic improvement beyond the early postinjection period, with greater improvements in pain and functional scores reported at midterm follow-up compared to corticosteroids.[42] Systematic reviews and guideline-based evaluations have concluded that while PRP may offer longer lasting symptom relief in some patients, current evidence does not demonstrate consistent or clinically meaningful superiority over corticosteroid injections.

Platelet-rich Plasma versus Hyaluronic Acid

HA represents another widely used injectable therapy for knee OA. Given its widespread adoption, HA has served as a common comparator in clinical trials evaluating new biologic therapies such as PRP. RCTs have shown similar outcomes between the 2 therapies. Filardo and colleagues[43] conducted one of the earliest RCTs to compare the 2 injectables and found that both PRP and HA led to a statistically significant improvement in knee function and symptomatic relief; however, PRP injections were associated with greater acute swelling and pain postinjection. Moreover, Cole and colleagues[38] performed a double-blind RCT evaluating the efficacy of the 2 injectables and found no statistically significant differences in their primary outcome measure (WOMAC scores) at 4 timepoints within a year postinjection. This study did find that there was, however, a trend toward significance in the level of reduction in IL-1β and TNF-α biochemical levels in the PRP group, suggesting its potentially greater anti-inflammatory properties. In contrast to these individual trials, a meta-analysis incorporating 26 RCTs with over 2400 patients, demonstrated significantly greater improvements in pain and functional outcomes early following PRP, while reporting no significant difference in adverse events between the 2 treatments, thereby suggesting a potential advantage of PRP over HA.[44]

IMAGING AND STRUCTURAL EFFECTS

The potential disease-modifying effect on articular cartilage of PRP remains a subject of ongoing investigation. As symptomatic improvement does not necessarily correlate with structural preservation, objective imaging-based assessment is essential. Conventional radiography is the primary imaging modality for monitoring OA progression; however, lacks sensitivity for early or subtle structural changes.[45] MRI, while more expensive, allows for direct visualization of cartilage, synovium, and subchondral bone.[46] MRI assessment includes morphologic measures (semiquantitative scoring; quantitative cartilage volume/thickness) and compositional analysis (evaluating biochemical changes in proteoglycans and collagen).[45] Both techniques have demonstrated reliability for evaluating outcomes following PRP therapy.[46]

Current imaging evidence regarding structural benefits of PRP is conflicting.[47–53] Several studies, including randomized trials comparing PRP to HA or saline, have reported no significant structural benefits regarding Kellgren-Lawrence progression, cartilage thickness, or volume loss.[47–49] However, Bansal and colleagues[48] noted that while cartilage thickness did not increase, a higher proportion of PRP-treated patients demonstrated stable cartilage thickness compared to HA, suggesting a chondroprotective, disease slowing effect as opposed to a cartilage regenerative effect.

Conversely, other data support structure improvement.[51,52] Lisi and colleagues[51] demonstrated reduced articular damage on MRI in the PRP group compared with HA group. Raeissadat and colleagues[52] found that PRP combined with exercise therapy resulted in superior improvements in patellofemoral cartilage volume and synovitis on MRI compared with exercise therapy alone. Additionally, quantitative MRI techniques have detected potential improvements in cartilage composition even in the absence of morphologic changes.[53]

The discordance in the literature of structural benefits of PRP likely reflects the heterogeneity of PRP formulations and the limitations of current imaging data. Most studies are restricted by short-term follow-up, which may be insufficient to detect meaningful structural challenges in a chronic, slow-progressing disease like OA. Furthermore, there are numerous different MRI acquisition protocols, which makes comparison between studies difficult and may also contribute to variable outcomes in the literature.

SAFETY AND TOLERABILITY

Intra-articular PRP injections have demonstrated a favorable safety and tolerability profile across published clinical studies. Most adverse events reported are mild and self-limiting, typically consisting of transient postinjection pain, swelling, stiffness, or local discomfort within the first few days following treatment.[38,43] These reactions are generally attributed to the inflammatory response triggered by platelet activation and increased cytokine release rather than to infectious or toxic effects. Serious adverse effects, including a knee joint infection or prolonged synovitis, are rare and occur at rates comparable to other intra-articular injection therapies.[54]

When compared with corticosteroid injections, PRP appears to offer a similarly low short-term complication rate but without the theoretic risks associated with repeated corticosteroid exposure. Corticosteroids have been associated with potential chondrotoxicity, suppression of cartilage repair mechanisms, and accelerated structural progression when used frequently, particularly in patients with early stage disease.[41] In contrast, PRP, as an autologous product, avoids risks related to immunogenic reactions and systemic side effects, although postinjection inflammatory flare-ups may be more pronounced than those seen with corticosteroids.[43,54]

From a practical perspective, adherence to strict aseptic technique, appropriate patient counseling regarding expected symptoms postinjection, and avoidance of nonsteroidal anti-inflammatory medications in the peri-injection period are important considerations to optimize safety and treatment response. Despite its overall favorable safety profile, the lack of standardization in PRP preparation and administration remains a concern and underscores the necessity for consistent protocols and clinician experience when offering this treatment.[55]

PATIENT SELECTION AND CLINICAL APPLICATION

Appropriate patient selection appears to be a critical determinant of clinical outcomes following PRP therapy. The current body of evidence suggests that patients with mild-to-moderate knee OA derive the greatest symptomatic benefit, whereas those with advanced radiographic disease tend to experience more modest and less durable improvements.[43] Younger patients, those with lower body mass index (BMI), and individuals with higher baseline activity levels have also been reported to demonstrate more favorable responses to PRP treatment, although findings across studies are not entirely consistent.[54]

Disease severity plays a particularly important role in guiding clinical decision-making. PRP may be best positioned as a treatment option aimed at symptom modification and functional improvement rather than an alternative to surgical intervention in advanced OA. In this context, PRP is increasingly considered as part of a stepwise, nonoperative treatment algorithm rather than a standalone solution.[56]

Injection protocols vary widely across studies, with regimens ranging from a single injection to a series of 2 or 3 injections administered over several weeks. While some evidence suggests that multiple-injection protocols may provide more sustained symptom relief, no consensus has been established regarding the optimal number of injections or treatment intervals.[57] This variability complicates direct comparisons between studies and highlights the need for standardization guidelines further.

Clinically, PRP may be used either as a standalone injectable or as an adjunct to other conservative measures, including physical therapy, weight management and activity modification. Combination approaches, such as PRP with HA or structured rehabilitation programs, have also been explored, although evidence supporting their routine use remains limited.[56,58] Ultimately, individualized treatment decisions based on patient characteristics, expectations and disease stage remain essential when considering PRP for knee OA.

PRP represents a biologically plausible and increasingly utilized treatment option for knee OA, supported by a growing body of preclinical and clinical evidence. Current data suggest that PRP can provide meaningful symptomatic relief in selected patients, particularly those with mild-to-moderate arthrosis. However, the clinical effectiveness of PRP remains variable, reflecting substantial heterogeneity in patient selection, PRP preparation methods, injection protocols, and outcome assessment across studies. Importantly, there is currently no consistent high-quality evidence demonstrating PRP to be more effective than corticosteroid injections, particularly when cost and accessibility are considered. While comparative trials and meta-analyses indicate potential advantages of PRP over traditional injectable therapies in certain contexts, definitive superiority has not been consistently demonstrated, and its disease modifying potential remains uncertain. In addition, given its higher direct costs, PRP may be more appropriately considered in patients with mild-to-moderate OA who have failed or derived limited benefit from corticosteroid or HA injections and who wish to delay or avoid surgical intervention, rather than a first-line injectable therapy. As such, PRP should be viewed as an adjunct within a stepwise, nonoperative treatment strategy rather than a replacement for established therapies or surgical intervention in advanced disease.

Future research should prioritize standardized PRP formulations, clearly defined treatment protocols, and longer term follow-up incorporating both clinical and structural outcomes. Improved stratification of patient populations most likely to benefit from PRP will be essential to clarify its optimal role in the management of knee OA. Notably major professional societies including the American Association of Hip and Knee Surgeons and the American Academy of Orthopedic Surgeons do not endorse the routine use of PRP injections for knee OA, reflecting the ongoing uncertainty surrounding its comparative efficacy, cost-effectiveness, and lack of standardized preparation methods.[59,60]

CLINICS CARE POINTS

- PRP may provide symptomatic improvement in selected patients with mild-to-moderate knee OA, but outcomes are variable.
- Patient selection is critical: younger patients, lower BMI, and earlier stage disease are more likely to benefit.
- PRP should be used as an adjunct within a stepwise nonoperative strategy, not as a replacement for established therapies or surgery.
- There is no standardized PRP formulation or protocol, limiting reproducibility and interpretation of outcomes.
- PRP has a favorable safety profile, but patients should be counseled regarding postinjection inflammatory flare.

FUNDING

This research did not receive any specific grant from funding agencies in the public, commercial, or not-for-profit sectors.

DISCLOSURE

Competing Interest: W. Wignadasan, T. Chae, M.E. Neufeld, L.C. Howard, and B.A. Masri do not receive any financial support and do not have any conflicts of interest.

REFERENCES

1. Scott CEH, Holland G, Krahelski O, et al. Patterns of cartilage loss and anterior cruciate ligament status in end-stage osteoarthritis of the knee. Bone Joint J 2020;102-B(6):716–26.
2. Collaborators GO. Global, regional, and national burden of osteoarthritis, 1990-2020 and projections to 2050: a systematic analysis for the global burden of disease study 2021. Lancet Rheumatol 2023;5(9):e508–22.
3. Hunter DJ, Bierma-Zeinstra S. Osteoarthritis. Lancet 2019;393(10182):1745–59.
4. Wijn SRW, Rovers MM, van Tienen TG, et al. Intra-articular corticosteroid injections increase the risk of requiring knee arthroplasty. Bone Joint J 2020;102-B(5):586–92.
5. Rutjes AW, Jüni P, da Costa BR, et al. Viscosupplementation for osteoarthritis of the knee: a systematic review and meta-analysis. Ann Intern Med 2012;157(3):180–91.
6. Boswell SG, Cole BJ, Sundman EA, et al. Platelet-rich plasma: a milieu of bioactive factors. Arthroscopy 2012;28(3):429–39.
7. Mazzocca AD, McCarthy MB, Chowaniec DM, et al. Platelet-rich plasma differs according to preparation method and human variability. J Bone Joint Surg Am 2012;94(4):308–16.
8. Sundman EA, Cole BJ, Fortier LA. Growth factor and catabolic cytokine concentrations are influenced by the cellular composition of platelet-rich plasma. Am J Sports Med 2011;39(10):2135–40.
9. Moussa M, Lajeunesse D, Hilal G, et al. Platelet rich plasma (PRP) induces chondroprotection via increasing autophagy, anti-inflammatory markers, and decreasing apoptosis in human osteoarthritic cartilage. Exp Cell Res 2017;352(1):146–56.
10. Lewis E, Merghani K, Robertson I, et al. The effectiveness of leucocyte-poor platelet-rich plasma injections on symptomatic early osteoarthritis of the knee: the PEAK randomized controlled trial. Bone Joint J 2022;104-B(6):663–71.
11. Belk JW, Kraeutler MJ, Houck DA, et al. Platelet-rich plasma versus hyaluronic acid for knee osteoarthritis: a systematic review and meta-analysis of randomized controlled trials. Am J Sports Med 2021;49(1):249–60.
12. Boffa A, Moraca G, Sangiorgio A, et al. Corticosteroids versus platelet-rich plasma injections for knee osteoarthritis: where is there more evidence? A systematic review of 60 years of literature. Knee 2025;55:104–11.
13. Khalid S, Ali A, Deepak F, et al. Comparative effectiveness of intra-articular therapies in knee osteoarthritis: a meta-analysis comparing platelet-rich plasma (PRP) with other treatment modalities. Ann Med Surg 2024;86(1):361–72.

14. Xie X, Zhang C, Tuan RS. Biology of platelet-rich plasma and its clinical application in cartilage repair. Arthritis Res Ther 2014;16(1):204.
15. Xu J, Chen X, Zhang H, et al. Platelet-rich plasma relieves inflammation and pain by regulating M1/M2 macrophage polarization in knee osteoarthritis rats. Sci Rep 2025;15(1):12805.
16. Choi M-C, Jo J, Park J, et al. NF-κB signaling pathways in osteoarthritic cartilage destruction. Cells 2019;8(7):734.
17. Wang K, Luo H, Liu L, et al. Frontiers | blockade of IL-1 family cytokines in the treatment of rheumatoid arthritis. Front Pharmacol 2025;16:1577628.
18. Bendinelli P, Matteucci E, Dogliotti G, et al. Molecular basis of anti-inflammatory action of platelet-rich plasma on human chondrocytes: mechanisms of NF-κB inhibition via HGF. J Cell Physiol 2010;225(3):757–66.
19. Fitzpatrick J, Bulsara MK, McCrory PR, et al. Analysis of platelet-rich plasma extraction. Orthop J Sports Med 2017;5(1):2325967116675272.
20. Dohan Ehrenfest DM, Rasmusson L, Albrektsson T. Classification of platelet concentrates: from pure platelet-rich plasma (P-PRP) to leucocyte- and platelet-rich fibrin (L-PRF) - PubMed. Trends Biotechnol 2009;27(3):158–67.
21. DeLong JM, Russell RP, Mazzocca AD. Platelet-rich plasma: the PAW classification system. Arthroscopy 2012;28(7):998–1009.
22. Mautner J, Malanga GA, Smith J, et al. A call for a standard classification system for future biologic research: the rationale for new PRP nomenclature. PM & R 2015;7(4 Suppl):S53–9.
23. Magalon J, Chateau AL, Bertrand B, et al. DEPA classification: a proposal for standardising PRP use and a retrospective application of available devices. BMJ 2016;2(1):e000060.
24. Lana JFSD, Purita J, Paulus C, et al. Contributions for classification of platelet rich plasma – proposal of a new classification: MARSPILL. Regen Med 2017;12(5):565–74.
25. Collins T, Alexander D, Barkatali B. Platelet-rich plasma: a narrative review. EFORT Open Rev 2021;6(4):225–35.
26. Braun HJ, Kim HJ, Chu CR, et al. The effect of platelet-rich plasma formulations and blood products on human synoviocytes: implications for intra-articular injury and therapy. Am J Sports Med 2014;42(5):1204–10.
27. Martino AD, Boffa A, Andriolo L, et al. Leukocyte-rich versus leukocyte-poor platelet-rich plasma for the treatment of knee osteoarthritis: a double-blind randomized trial. Am J Sports Med 2022;50(3):609–17.
28. Kim J-H, Park Y-B, Ha C-W, et al. Adverse reactions and clinical outcomes for leukocyte-poor versus leukocyte-rich platelet-rich plasma in knee osteoarthritis: a systematic review and meta-analysis. Orthop J Sports Med 2021;9(6):23259671211011948.
29. L Y, L Z, D X, et al. Chondroprotective effects of platelet lysate towards monoiodoacetate-induced arthritis by suppression of TNF-α-induced activation of NF-κB pathway in chondrocytes. Aging 2019;11(9):2797–811.
30. Bensa A, Previtali D, Sangiorgio A, et al. PRP injections for the treatment of knee osteoarthritis: the improvement is clinically significant and influenced by platelet concentration: a meta-analysis of randomized controlled trials. Am J Sports Med 2025;53(3):745–54.
31. Simental-Mendía M, Acosta-Olivo CA, Ortega-Mata D, et al. Influence of platelet count on the clinical effectiveness of platelet-rich plasma in the treatment of knee osteoarthritis: a systematic review and meta-analysis. Orthopaedics & Traumatology: Surgery & Research 2025;104453.
32. Foster TE, Puskas BL, Mandelbaum BR, et al. Platelet-rich plasma. Am J Sports Med 2009;37(11):2259–72.
33. Cavallo C, Roffi A, Grigolo B, et al. Platelet-rich plasma: the choice of activation method affects the release of bioactive molecules. BioMed Res Int 2016;2016:6591717.
34. Simental-Mendía M, Ortega-Mata D, Tamez-Mata Y, et al. Comparison of the clinical effectiveness of activated and non-activated platelet-rich plasma in the treatment of knee osteoarthritis: a systematic review and meta-analysis. Clin Rheumatol 2022;42(5):1397–408.
35. Patel S, Dhillon MS, Aggarwal S, et al. Treatment with platelet-rich plasma is more effective than placebo for knee osteoarthritis: a prospective, double-blind, randomized trial. Am J Sports Med 2013;41(2):356–64.
36. Görmeli G, Görmeli CA, Ataoglu B, et al. Multiple PRP injections are more effective than single injections and hyaluronic acid in knees with early osteoarthritis: a randomized, double-blind, placebo-controlled trial. Knee Surg Sports Traumatol Arthrosc 2017;25(3):958–65.
37. Dai WL, Zhou AG, Zhang H, et al. Efficacy of platelet-rich plasma in the treatment of knee osteoarthritis: a meta-analysis of randomized controlled trials. Arthroscopy 2017;33(3):659–70.e1.
38. Cole BJ, Karas V, Hussey K, et al. Hyaluronic acid versus platelet-rich plasma: a prospective, double-blind randomized controlled trial comparing clinical outcomes and effects on intra-articular biology for the treatment of knee osteoarthritis. Am J Sports Med 2017;45(2):339–46.
39. Campbell KA, Saltzman BM, Mascarenhas R, et al. Does intra-articular platelet-rich plasma injection provide clinically superior outcomes compared

with other therapies in the treatment of knee osteoarthritis? A systematic review of overlapping meta-analyses. Arthroscopy 2015;31(11):2213–21.

40. Bennell KL, Paterson KL, Metcalf BR, et al. Effect of intra-articular platelet-rich plasma vs placebo injection on pain and medial tibial cartilage volume in patients with knee osteoarthritis: the RESTORE randomized clinical trial. JAMA 2021;326(20):2021–30.
41. McAlindon TE, LaValley MP, Harvey WF, et al. Effect of intra-articular triamcinolone vs saline on knee cartilage volume and pain in patients with knee osteoarthritis: a randomized clinical trial. JAMA 2017;317(19):1967–75.
42. Huang Y, Liu X, Xu X, et al. Intra-articular injections of platelet-rich plasma, hyaluronic acid or corticosteroids for knee osteoarthritis : a prospective randomized controlled study. Orthopä 2019;48(3):239–47.
43. Filardo G, Di Matteo B, Di Martino A, et al. Platelet-rich plasma intra-articular knee injections show no superiority versus viscosupplementation: a randomized controlled trial. Am J Sports Med 2015; 43(7):1575–82.
44. Tan J, Chen H, Zhao L, et al. Platelet-rich plasma versus hyaluronic acid in the treatment of knee osteoarthritis: a meta-analysis of 26 randomized controlled trials. Arthroscopy 2021;37(1):309–25.
45. Roemer FW, Guermazi A, Demehri S, et al. Imaging in osteoarthritis. Osteoarthr Cartil 2022;30(7).
46. Hunter DJ, Zhang W, Conaghan PG, et al. Responsiveness and reliability of MRI in knee osteoarthritis: a meta-analysis of published evidence. Osteoarthr Cartil 2011;19(5):589–605.
47. Buendía-López D, Medina-Quirós M, Fernández-Villacañas Marín MÁ. Clinical and radiographic comparison of a single LP-PRP injection, a single hyaluronic acid injection and daily NSAID administration with a 52-week follow-up: a randomized controlled trial. J Orthop Traumatol 2018;19(1):3.
48. Bansal H, Leon J, Pont JL, et al. Platelet-rich plasma (PRP) in osteoarthritis (OA) knee: correct dose critical for long term clinical efficacy. Sci Rep 2021; 11(1):3971.
49. Bennell KL, Paterson KL, Metcalf BR, et al. Effect of intra-articular platelet-rich plasma vs placebo on pain and cartilage volume in knee osteoarthritis. JAMA 2021;326(20):2021–30.
50. Sax OC, Chen Z, Mont MA, et al. The efficacy of platelet-rich plasma for the treatment of knee osteoarthritis symptoms and structural changes: a systematic review and meta-analysis. J Arthroplast 2022;37(11):2282–90.e2.
51. Lisi C, Perotti C, Scudeller L, et al. Treatment of knee osteoarthritis: platelet-derived growth factors vs. hyaluronic acid. A randomized controlled trial. Clin Rehabil 2018;32(3):330–9.
52. Raeissadat SA, Ghorbani E, Taheri MS, et al. MRI changes after platelet rich plasma injection in knee osteoarthriti | JPR. J Pain Res 2020;13:65–73.
53. Tschopp M, Pfirrmann CWA, Brunner F, et al. Morphological and quantitative parametric MRI Follow-up of cartilage changes before and after intra-articular injection therapy in patients with mild to moderate knee osteoarthritis: a randomized, placebo-controlled trial. Investig Radiol 2024;59(9): 646–55.
54. Andia I, Maffulli N. Platelet-rich plasma for managing pain and inflammation in osteoarthritis. Nat Rev Rheumatol 2013;9(12):721–30.
55. Dohan EDM, Andia I, Zumstein MA, et al. Classification of platelet concentrates (Platelet-Rich Plasma-PRP, platelet-rich Fibrin-PRF) for topical and infiltrative use in orthopedic and sports medicine: current consensus, clinical implications and perspectives. Muscles Ligaments Tendons J 2014; 4(1):3–9.
56. Bannuru RR, Osani MC, Vaysbrot EE, et al. OARSI guidelines for the non-surgical management of knee, hip, and polyarticular osteoarthritis. Osteoarthr Cartil 2019;27(11):1578–89.
57. Laudy AB, Bakker EW, Rekers M, et al. Efficacy of platelet-rich plasma injections in osteoarthritis of the knee: a systematic review and meta-analysis. Br J Sports Med 2015;49(10):657–72.
58. Ciapini G, Simonettii M, Giuntoli M, et al. Is the combination of platelet-rich plasma and hyaluronic acid the best injective treatment for grade II-III knee osteoarthritis? A prospective study. Adv Orthop 2023;2023:1868943.
59. Surgeons AAoHaK. Biologics for advanced hip and knee arthritis. 2025. Available at: https://www.aahks.org/position-statements/biologics-for-advanced-hip-and-knee-arthritis/.
60. Surgeons AAoO. Platelet-rich plasma <h3 data-end="840: data-start="819">. 2025. Available at: https://orthoinfo.aaos.org/en/treatment/platelet-rich-plasma-prp/.

Advances in Gene Therapy for Osteoarthritis

A Review of the Literature

J. Michael Ruth Jr, MD, William M. Mihalko, MD, PhD*, Christopher Holland, MD, MS

KEYWORDS

• Osteoarthritis • Gene therapy • Cartilage degeneration • Cytokines • Viral vectors

KEY POINTS

- Osteoarthritis is a complex disease process with many contributing factors, ranging from genetic to environmental.
- New research has identified mechanisms through which genetics influence the development and progression of osteoarthritis.
- Advancements in gene therapy technology have made it possible for the development of disease-modifying osteoarthritis drugs that target these mechanisms.
- Future advances in gene therapy could provide viable treatment and prevention options for patients who are unable to undergo arthroplasty.

INTRODUCTION

Background/Epidemiology

Osteoarthritis (OA) is one of the most ubiquitous diseases worldwide, affecting around 500 million people or 7% of the global population.[1] Between 1990 and 2019, the number of people affected by OA globally increased by 48%, resulting in it being the 15th-ranked cause of years lived with disability.[1] In the United States alone, at least 33 million adults have OA and around 14 million of those have symptomatic knee arthritis.[2,3] Typically, OA is thought of as a disease that disproportionately affects the elderly; however, approximately 2 million people under age 45 and 6 million people 45 to 64 year old suffer from it.[3] As the prevalence of hip and knee OA has increased, especially in younger demographics, the overall burden on quality of life has increased substantially.[4] This has led to patients seeking total joint arthroplasty earlier in their lives.[4,5] The number of patients undergoing total joint arthroplasty, especially those younger than 65 years of age, has dramatically increased, thought to be in part to the rise of obesity and an aging population.[5] In 2000, approximately 6% of Americans had symptomatic knee OA and 3% had symptomatic hip OA.[6] By 2012, approximately 22.7% of all Americans had OA.[7] This is projected to increase to approximately 26% of all Americans by 2040 with 11.4% of all adults having an arthritis-attributable activity limitation.[7] The demographics of joint replacement patients have changed over the years as implants have improved. Many joint replacement patients nowadays are more educated, more active, and physiologically younger than were seen previously.[8] Physical and mental health are associated with patient function and mobility.[9] As such, patients with symptomatic OA have been shown to have higher odds of developing depression, coronary heart disease, and even

University of Tennessee Health Science Center-Campbell Clinic, Department of Orthopaedic Surgery and Biomedical Engineering, Memphis, TN, USA
* Corresponding author. University of Tennessee Health Science Center-Campbell Clinic, Department of Orthopaedic Surgery and Biomedical Engineering, 956 Court Avenue, Memphis, TN 38103.
E-mail address: wmihalko@campbellclinic.com

Orthop Clin N Am 57 (2026) 307–316
https://doi.org/10.1016/j.ocl.2026.05.003

Abbreviations	
AAV	adeno-associated virus
ACC	articular chondrocyte
DAMP	damage-associated molecular pattern
DMOAD	disease-modifying osteoarthritis drug
EC	early chondrocyte
ECM	extracellular matrix
GPC	growth plate chondrocyte
miRNA	micro RNA
MMP	matrix metalloproteinase
OA	osteoarthritis
PRR	pattern recognition receptor
SSC	skeletogenic stem cell

higher all-cause mortality compared to their nonarthritic peers.[10–13] Improved treatment options exist nowadays, but overall patient satisfaction status after surgical or nonsurgical treatment is not yet approaching 100%. New therapies that address the underlying biochemical and genetic mechanisms that contribute to the development of this disease could significantly improve patient satisfaction, decrease morbidity, and potentially result in overall lower healthcare spending globally.

Normal Cartilage Biology

Articular cartilage is a highly specialized tissue with a principal function of providing a smooth lubricated surface for articulation and allowing for transmission of loads.[14] It is a 2- to 4-mm thick layer of hyaline cartilage comprised of an extracellular matrix (ECM) of collagen, water, and proteoglycans, and chondrocytes which function to build and maintain the ECM.[15,16] Chondrocytes develop from mesenchymal multipotent skeletogenic stem cells (SSCs). These SSCs then undergo further growth and differentiation into growth plate chondrocytes (GPCs) or articular chondrocytes (ACCs) which become bone via endochondral ossification and articular cartilage, respectfully.[17] SSCs undergo differentiation into early chondrocytes (ECs) via the SOX9 transcription factor which instructs them to express genes like COL1A1, COL2A1, and ACAN to produce copious ECM. SOX 9 can be thought of as the EC master transcription factor, whereas further differentiation into GPCs is driven by RUNX2/3 and ACCs by RELA. The expression of RUNX2/3 results in ECM production and facilitates alignment of the chondrocytes into columns. These columnar chondrocytes then express Indian hedgehog and WNT5a which stimulate proliferation/maturation and alignment, respectively. In ACCs, RELA activation drives chondrocyte proliferation and ECM assembly. Unlike GPCs, ACC maturation is much simpler. Due to the lack of collagen turnover for endochondral ossification, only the aggrecans undergo turnover.[17–19] When ACCs reach maturity they secrete lubricin, encoded by the PRG4 gene.[17] This glycoprotein has multiple functions in promoting overall health and function of articular cartilage. Acting as a boundary lubricant, lubricin reduces friction between the 2 articular surfaces thus decreasing the incidence of chondrocyte cell death in the more superficial layers of cartilage.[20,21] Lubricin has also been shown to decrease synovial membrane hyperplasia, decrease chondrocyte apoptosis, and help to facilitate synovial cell proliferation and adhesion.[20–23] Patients with OA have been shown to have decreased levels of lubricin expression and subsequent supplementation has resulted in symptom improvement.[20] While lubricin has primarily been shown to be protective, when it is found in inflamed arthritic tissue it can carry a ligand responsible for leukocyte recruitment, potentially furthering the development of OA.[24] Overall, the literature reports lubricin as a functional marker for the presence of healthy articular cartilage and treatments that work by preservation or supplementation of this glycoprotein help to improve overall patient function.

Pathogenesis/Pathophysiology of Osteoarthritis

OA is driven by the breakdown of articular cartilage. This destruction results in uneven or rough articular surfaces and subsequent osteophyte and bone cyst formation with areas of sclerosis close to the joint line. Early stages of OA show proteoglycan depletion and collagen disarray. As it progresses, the later stages are characterized by significant losses in collagen, water content, and proteoglycans resulting in significant disruption of articular cartilage's ability to distribute loads.[25]

The pathophysiology of OA is multifactorial. A noninclusive list of these risk factors includes aging, mechanical stress, hereditary causes, inflammation, metabolism, and trauma.[23,25] As patients age, they acquire age-related modifications in their mitochondrial DNA due to accumulated mutations and long-term exposure to oxidative stress. This dysfunction results in the excessive generation of reactive oxygen species and resultant oxidative damage and cell death via inflammatory response activation. This progressive decline in chondrocyte population results in exacerbated joint dysfunction and OA progression.[25]

Mechanical stress can contribute to apoptosis of chondrocytes through several different pathways. While some mechanical loading is necessary for cartilage health as it stimulates proteoglycan production, excess loading due to increased body weight from obesity accelerates cartilage wear and drives osteophyte production.[25–27] Excessive articular cartilage loading drives reactive oxygen species (ROS) release from mitochondria, resulting in chondrocyte cell death and ECM degradation. These damaged chondrocytes release alarmins and other proinflammatory cytokines that drive inflammation and further cartilage loss.[28]

Hereditary mutations in genes encoding collagen proteins, inflammatory markers, hormone receptor proteins, growth factors such as IGF-1 and TGF-b, metalloproteases, and BMPs have been shown to play a role in the development of OA.[29] Newer research has also shown that micro RNAs (miRNAs), small single-stranded RNA molecules, can have a significant impact on the pathogenesis of OA. These molecules function by repressing translation or degrading specific messenger RNAs to regulate post-transcriptional gene expression. Several have been identified and generally have been found to have increased or decreased levels in osteoarthritic patients. MiR-9-5p, for example, is associated with suppressing chondrocyte apoptosis and has a protective role against the development of OA. Its levels are decreased in patients with OA. Other miRNAs that have been found to play a pathologic role in OA are miR-485-5p and miR-146a-5p, which inhibit MSC differentiation into chondroblasts and increase cartilage degradation via inflammation, respectively.[30]

Inflammation is a significant factor in the pathogenesis of OA. Traditionally OA was not thought to be an inflammatory-driven process, but as our understanding of the disease has progressed, it has been found to be a central pillar of its progression. Inflammatory processes drive catabolic changes in the cartilage matrix via matrix metalloproteinases (MMPs), aggrecanases, and other degradative enzymes as well as antianabolic effects in chondrocytes.[23,31] Furthermore, the school of thought that OA is simply a disease of articular cartilage is falling out of favor. While it is true that the mainstay of OA is the progressive degeneration of articular cartilage, the disease affects the entire joint.[31] The inflammation in OA differs from a true inflammatory arthritis in the fact that it is a low-grade response primarily driven by the innate immune system. Injury to the joint, acute, chronic, or otherwise, and the resulting tissue breakdown results in activation of pattern recognition receptors (PRRs) by damage-associated molecular patterns (DAMPs) and subsequent macrophage and mast cell activation and production of inflammatory cytokines.[32] The cytokines most implicated are tumor necrosis factor (TNF) alpha, interleukin (IL)-1b, IL-6, IL-1Ra, IL-10, which promote osteoarthritic changes to articular cartilage by directing chondrocytes to synthesize MMPs, aggrecanases, proteases, chemokines, nitric oxide, leukotrienes, and prostaglandins.[32–34] MMPs function to break down both the structural backbone (type II collagen) and proteoglycans in the ECM. In OA, ADAMTS-4 and ADAMTS-5 are the primary enzymes responsible for aggrecan degradation and MMP-13 is the primary enzyme responsible for collagen degradation.[35] These proteinases and inflammatory cytokines work together to drive catabolic effects and anti-anabolic effects on articular cartilage and create an overall picture of synovitis affecting the entire joint.[36]

Metabolism plays a unique role in the pathogenesis of OA. There is increasing evidence that OA is a metabolic disorder and that aberrant metabolism in chondrocytes, synoviocytes, and osteocytes directly contributes to the production of inflammatory cytokines and chemokines.[37–39] Obesity and type 2 diabetes are 2 metabolic conditions that are known risk factors for OA. Obesity provides both mechanical and inflammatory insults to the joint. Excessive cumulative mechanical contact stress due to high body weight causes chondrocyte cell death from excess loading and adipokines secreted by adipocytes trigger systemic inflammation, protease activation, and chondrocyte degradation. Type 2 diabetes further compounds this picture through metabolic reprogramming, resulting in subsequent cellular senescence and OA.[28,31,40]

Trauma contributes to the pathogenesis of OA through both mechanical and inflammatory mechanisms. Mechanical damage results in acute cell death and gross change to the joint structure as well as release of DAMPs which through PRRs initiate an inflammatory cascade and the resultant activation of catabolic pathways and enzymes as described above[28,41]

Current Treatment Options

Because OA is a multifactorial disease, there are many different potential targets for treatment. Currently, however, the standard of care can be broken down into 2 categories: conservative/medical management and surgical management. Medical management typically consists of oral anti-inflammatory medications, intra-articular glucocorticoid injections, visco supplementation, weight loss, and physical therapy. The mainstay of surgical OA management is arthroplasty.[42–45] Newer treatment options that use small molecule drugs or neutralizing antibodies to target specific inflammatory processes are currently in clinical trial, but despite our newfound understanding of the disease treatment satisfaction rates are not great.[46] In fact, patient satisfaction with nonoperative treatment has been shown to be around 68% and surgical treatment with total knee arthroplasty (TKA) only affords 80% to 85% satisfaction.[47,48] Gene therapy is a new treatment option that aims to provide lasting treatment options for patients with minimal side effects due to the extreme specificity of their mechanism.

GENE THERAPY TO TREAT OSTEOARTHRITIS

Basic Overview

Gene therapy has been proposed as treatment for OA for around 20 years as a solution to promote sustained local production of promotors of cartilage repair such as TGF-b, IGF, and BMP.[49] Synovial cells readily accept genes via both viral and non-viral vectors. Using these vectors for facilitating prolonged transgene expression is a beneficial trait to have for the treatment of chronic disease. Proof of concept for gene therapy has been demonstrated for some time now. Studies using animal models have shown the efficacy of an adenovirus-based gene therapy to increase expression of the cartilage-protective IL-1Ra protein since 2004, and China has been using a gene therapy to treat head and neck cancer since 2003.[50,51] Gene therapies work by utilizing a vector to transfer genes of interest into host cells. These genes are typically in the form of cDNAs and are transferred into host cells in a way that facilitates nuclear translocation and high transgene expression. While there are other types of vectors, traditionally viruses have been utilized due to their innate ability to effectively translocate their own genome. When choosing a virus to use as a vector, it is important to remove the sequences that contribute to virulence and disease while maintaining its ability to infect cells. Safety considerations center around whether the vector integrates its genome into the host cell (which can cause cancer) and if it causes unintentional immune responses which can result in limited transgene expression and systemic inflammatory complications.[52–55] Viral vectors can deliver gene therapy in-vivo, or ex-vivo. In-vivo vectors are introduced directly into the body whereas ex-vivo vectors are introduced into cells that are then subsequently placed into the injury site.[51] Ex-vivo therapy works in concert with tissue engineering, as the implantation of tissues has the potential to physically restore the damage and then protects the repair from degradation using transgene expression. However, it is significantly more costly than in-vivo therapy.[56,57] Non-viral mechanisms can prevent some of these potential issues and the development of biomaterials as vectors has shown promising results.[58]

Targets for Gene Therapy

The multitude of inflammatory cytokines, transcription factors, enzymes, and regulatory molecules lends many targets for a gene therapy approach to treatment.[57,59] The goal of this treatment approach is to upregulate therapeutic genes and downregulate deleterious genes. As such, most research has primarily focused on the modulation of proinflammatory and anti-inflammatory cytokines due to their ease of modulation and their prominent contribution to the pathogenesis of OA.[57] Common cytokines targeted for gene therapy include IL-1Ra, IL-1b, IL-10, and IL-4.[57,60–62] Growth factors such as FGF-2, FGF-18, IGF-1, TGFb-1, and BMP-2 have also shown promise as potential targets.[57,60,63]

Transcription factors offer an even wider breadth of targets that range from extremely upstream in the expression pathway, such as SOX-9, to FLI1 and ERG which regulate specific protein expression.[17,19,57] Other potential transcription factor targets include RelA, the transcription factor that drives ACC differentiation, NFATC2 which drives RNF125 gene expression and is associated with inhibited ECM degradation, NFATC1 and 4 of which knockout mutations are associated with spontaneous OA development in mice, nuclear factor kappa-light-chain-enhancer of activated B cells (NF-kB) which drives HIF2a and 3a expression, both of which promote cartilage catabolism.[17,19,64–66] Heterozygous knockout mutations of the RelA transcription factor have also been shown to suppress OA development through inhibition of catabolic gene expression.[65] NKX3.2 is another transcription factor that has shown promise as a target for gene therapy as it can help protect chondrocytes from programmed cell death.[67–69]

Enzymes such as aggrecanases and proteinases can be targeted at several levels, from the protein itself to the transcription factors and genes that help encode them. For example, downregulating the Runx2 transcription factor can decrease the production of MMP-13, the main collagenase of OA.[57]

Viral-Based Mechanisms

The most common viruses used as vectors for gene therapy are adeno-associated viruses (AAVs), adenoviruses, retroviruses, and lentiviruses.[51,58] Baculoviruses have also been used as vectors for gene therapy targeting TGF-b1, IGF-1, and BMP-2 expression, but they do not replicate and this transgene expression typically occurs for less than 7 days. Adenoviruses, AAVs, and baculoviruses have a safety advantage over retro and lentiviruses since they do not integrate into the host genome. The downside to this is that transgene expression is markedly shorter with lenti/retroviruses showing sustained, long-term expression.[58] Currently, AAVs and lentiviruses have shown the most promise for use as vectors with lasting transgene expression, utility, and safety profile.[59] Of all viral vectors, recombinant AAV is thought of as the least toxic and results in the least induction of innate and adaptive immunity and can support transgene expression in-vivo for 10 years.[70] AAV 2, 5, 6, and 6.2 are the most efficient serotypes for transducing gene therapies into chondrocytes in the setting of OA.[71] Unfortunately, most adults display some seroprevalence of neutralizing antibodies to AAVs, with AAV 1 being the most prevalent and AAV 5 being the least prevalent.[71] Given this finding, AAV 5 appears to be the most ideal AAV vector for the delivery of gene therapies to chondrocytes.

AAV-based vectors have a proven track record for use in delivering gene therapies.[72–74] Most research using AAVs in the setting of OA has focused on an IL-1Ra-based therapy. Several groups have proved that targeting this pathway shows promising results for the development of a disease-modifying OA drug (DMOAD) demonstrated through small and large animal models and even efficacy for use in vertebral disc degeneration.[75–77] The most developed therapy focuses on sc-rAAV2.5IL-1Ra. This sc-rAAV2.5IL-1Ra therapy is administered via intra-articular injection and has shown proven efficacy in rat and equine models as well as safety and efficacy in human clinical trials.[78–81] Other AAV-based therapies have targeted transcription factors such as SOX9 and growth factors such as FGF-2 and IGF-1, and proteoglycan (lubricin) production with promising results.[82–85]

Nonviral Mechanisms

Nonviral based mechanisms include cell-based therapies, CRISPR/gene editing, miRNA (noncoding RNAs that regulate gene expression)-based therapies, engineered extracellular vesicles, sono/electroporation, lipid-based carriers, polymer-based carriers, and scaffold-based gene therapies.[56,58,86–90] By avoiding the use of viral vectors, there is less concern that the hosts' immune system will become sensitized and that humoral and adaptive immune responses will prevent transgene expression.

Cell-based therapies have demonstrated efficacy in treating OA symptoms safely. The most prominent cell therapy, TissueGene C (Kolon Tissuegene, Inc.), is an injectable therapy consisting of genetically engineered allogenic human chondrocytes that express TGF-B1, which has been shown to drive chondrocyte proliferation and proteoglycan production. These chondrocytes are derived from a single human donor and virally transduced via a retroviral vector to stimulate cartilage regeneration through cytokine production. These cells are then injected into the knee joint using a syringe. When compared to placebo in a multicenter, double-blinded, placebo-controlled, randomized study, this therapy was shown to have a significant improvement in knee function and decrease in pain at 12 weeks.[91] Further studies in humans have shown significant improvements in pain, stiffness, and motor function when compared to placebo demonstrated by Western Ontario and McMaster Universities Osteoarthritis Index (WOMAC), International Knee Documentation Committee (IKDC), and Visual Analog Scale (VAS) scores.[92] TissueGene C also has been shown to provide long-term analgesia through neuromodulation in a rat model, an additional potential method of symptom improvement.[93] No serious adverse events have occurred with human trials of this treatment and most side effects have been due to injection-site reactions.[92]

Gene editing is a novel new mechanism for the treatment of disease. As new research has shown that inflammation influences epigenetic factors through DNA methylation and demethylation, using therapies that affect gene expression have become a plausible means of OA treatment via prevention.[94] Using the CRISPR/Cas9 system to edit the genome, several potential targets for gene therapy have been identified. Induction of a knockout mutation in the IL1-R1 receptor gene (receptor for IL-1b) using the CRISPR/Cas9 system allowed human articular cartilage to become nonresponsive to the effects of IL-1b, one of the most potent inflammatory cytokines involved in the pathogenesis of OA.[95] An additional benefit of using a CRISPR/Cas9 system as opposed to a viral vector, is that it can be encapsulated in an extracellular vesicle derived from the chondrocyte mesenchymal stem cells preventing degradation in vivo by immune recognition and help facilitate transport to the target tissue.[96] Gene editing could also be utilized to address the cellular senescence associated with chondrocytes by upregulating CBX4, a protein associated with nucleolar homeostasis and gene expression. The overexpression of CBX4 has shown an ability to reduce human mesenchymal stem cell aging and alleviate the development of OA in mice.[96–98]

Therapies that target miRNAs, such as those affecting MiR-210 and MiR-140, are also potential avenues to explore regarding additional treatment options for OA. Decreased circulating MiR-210 has been shown to be associated with expression of proinflammatory cytokines related to the NF-KB pathway. Overexpression of this miRNA in a rat model resulted in decreased inflammation through the inhibition of NF-KB. MiR-140 expression has been shown to not only decrease inflammation through decreased expression of IL-1B, IL-6, IL-8 and downregulation of ADAMTS-5, but to also increase expression of ACAN, SOX9, and enzymes associated with the increased expression of chondroitin sulfate.[99–102] Intra-articular injections of MiR-140 in rats have been found to prevent the progression of OA through this mechanism of decreased MMP-13/ADAMTS-5 expression and upregulation of enzymes that promote expression of Type II collagen.[103] Future targets of investigation regarding miRNA therapy include mechanosensitive miRNAs associated with cartilage and subchondral bone remodeling.[104]

Current Clinical Trials

Several active clinical trials in the United States utilize gene-based therapies for treating OA. TissueGene-C is undergoing Phase III clinical trials for use in the knee. Other current clinical trials utilized AAV-based vectors, with one using nonviral plasmid DNA. Two phase I/II trials are studying the efficacy and safety of an IL-1Ra-based therapy. An additional trial is investigating the use of Nkx3.2-D2. XT-150, a gene therapy based on nonviral plasmid DNA targeting IL-10, is in Phase II/III trials. All current therapies under investigation are focused primarily on knee OA.[62,63]

SUMMARY

The development of new therapeutics for OA has a bright future. This current explosion in gene-based therapies is leading the charge toward better treatment and possible prevention of a debilitating disease that affects millions globally. Since OA depends on many different factors that can be addressed at several levels, a multitude of targets are available for the development of DMOADs. If the safety and efficacy of these therapies can be continually demonstrated through clinical trials, a paradigm shift in the way we treat OA is just over the horizon.

CLINICS CARE POINTS

- Osteoarthritis is a multifactorial disease. Understanding this helps to better counsel patients on their diagnosis and treatment options.
- Not all patients who undergo arthroplasty will be satisfied with their results.
- Clinical trials are currently underway for gene therapies to treat osteoarthritis. Patients who are interested have a potential opportunity to participate in trials.
- Gene therapy will afford patients who cannot undergo surgery a medical treatment option that addresses a cause of their disease process instead of masking the symptoms

DISCLOSURE

Dr W.M. Mihalko receives royalties from Aesculap AG and Elsevier, and is a paid consultant for Smith & Nephew, Pacira Pharmaceuticals Inc., and Ceramtec Inc. He is a board or committee member of ISTA, ASTM, Hip Society, Knee Society, AAHKS, Campbell Clinic Foundation, Orthopedic Clinics of North America, Journal of Arthroplasty, Journal of Orthopedic Research, Journal of Long-Term Use of Medical Implants, Bioengineering. Dr C.T. Holland is a paid consultant for Smith & Nephew Orthopaedics. Dr J.M. Ruth reports no conflicts of interest.

REFERENCES

1. Hunter DJ, March L, Chew M. Osteoarthritis in 2020 and beyond: a lancet commission. Lancet 2020;396(10264):1711–2.
2. .https://www.cdc.gov/arthritis/osteoarthritis/index.html.

3. Deshpande BR, Katz JN, Solomon DH, et al. Number of persons with symptomatic knee osteoarthritis in the US: impact of race and ethnicity, age, sex, and obesity. Arthritis Care Res (Hoboken) 2016;68(12):1743–50.
4. Ackerman IN, Bucknill A, Page RS, et al. The substantial personal burden experienced by younger people with hip or knee osteoarthritis. Osteoarthr Cartil 2015;23(8):1276–84.
5. Losina E, Thornhill TS, Rome BN, et al. The dramatic increase in total knee replacement utilization rates in the United States cannot be fully explained by growth in population size and the obesity epidemic. J Bone Joint Surg Am 2012; 94(3):201–7.
6. Felson DT, Lawrence RC, Dieppe PA, et al. Osteoarthritis: new insights. Part 1: the disease and its risk factors. Annals of Internal Medicine 2000; 133(8):635–46.
7. Hootman JM, Helmick CG, Barbour KE, et al. Updated projected prevalence of self-reported doctor-diagnosed arthritis and arthritis-attributable activity limitation among US adults, 2015-2040. Arthritis Rheumatol 2016;68(7):1582–7.
8. Crowninshield RD, Rosenberg AG, Sporer SM. Changing demographics of patients with total joint replacement. Clin Orthop Relat Res 2006; 443:266–72.
9. Vina ER, Kwoh CK. Epidemiology of osteoarthritis: literature update. Curr Opin Rheumatol 2018; 30(2):160–7.
10. Chung WS, Lin HH, Ho FM, et al. Risks of acute coronary syndrome in patients with osteoarthritis: a nationwide population-based cohort study. Clin Rheumatol 2016;35(11):2807–13.
11. Courties A, Sellam J, Maheu E, et al. Coronary heart disease is associated with a worse clinical outcome of hand osteoarthritis: a cross-sectional and longitudinal study. RMD Open 2017;3(1):e000344.
12. Veronese N, Stubbs B, Solmi M, et al. Association between lower limb osteoarthritis and incidence of depressive symptoms: data from the osteoarthritis initiative. Age Ageing 2017;46(3):470–6.
13. Kluzek S, Sanchez-Santos MT, Leyland KM, et al. Painful knee but not hand osteoarthritis is an independent predictor of mortality over 23 years follow-up of a population-based cohort of middle-aged women. Ann Rheum Dis 2016;75(10):1749–56.
14. Sophia Fox AJ, Bedi A, Rodeo SA. The basic science of articular cartilage: structure, composition, and function. Sports Health 2009;1(6):461–8.
15. Buckwalter JA, Hunzinker E, Rosenberg L, et al. Articular cartilage: composition and structure. In: Woo SLY, Buckwalter JA, editors. Injury and repair of the musculoskeletal soft tissues. Park Ridge (IL): American Academy of Orthopaedic Surgeons; 1988. p. 405–25.
16. Buckwalter JA, Mankin HJ. Articular cartilage: tissue design and chondrocyte-matrix interactions. Instr Course Lect 1998;47:477–86.
17. Liu CF, Samsa WE, Zhou G, et al. Transcriptional control of chondrocyte specification and differentiation. Semin Cell Dev Biol 2017;62:34–49.
18. Kronenberg HM. Developmental regulation of the growth plate. Nature 2003;423(6937):332–6.
19. Richard D, Pregizer S, Venkatasubramanian D, et al. Lineage-specific differences and regulatory networks governing human chondrocyte development. eLife 2023;12.
20. Watkins AR, Reesink HL. Lubricin in experimental and naturally occurring osteoarthritis: a systematic review. Osteoarthr Cartil 2020;28(10):1303–15.
21. Waller KA, Zhang LX, Elsaid KA, et al. Role of lubricin and boundary lubrication in the prevention of chondrocyte apoptosis. Proc Natl Acad Sci U S A 2013;110(15):5852–7.
22. Rhee DK, Marcelino J, Baker M, et al. The secreted glycoprotein lubricin protects cartilage surfaces and inhibits synovial cell overgrowth. J Clin Investig 2005;115(3):622–31.
23. Szychlinska MA, Leonardi R, Al-Qahtani M, et al. Altered joint tribology in osteoarthritis: reduced lubricin synthesis due to the inflammatory process. New horizons for therapeutic approaches. Ann Phys Rehabil Med 2016;59(3):149–56.
24. Estrella RP, Whitelock JM, Packer NH, et al. The glycosylation of human synovial lubricin: implications for its role in inflammation. Biochem J 2010;429(2):359–67.
25. Hiruthyaswamy SP, Bose A, Upadhyay A, et al. Molecular signaling pathways in osteoarthritis and biomaterials for cartilage regeneration: a review. Bioengineered 2025;16(1):2501880.
26. Jørgensen AEM, Kjær M, Heinemeier KM. The effect of aging and mechanical loading on the metabolism of articular cartilage. J Rheumatol 2017; 44(4):410–7. Epub 2017 Mar 1. PMID: 28250141.
27. Takahashi I, Takeda K, Matsuzaki T, et al. Reduction of knee joint load suppresses cartilage degeneration, osteophyte formation, and synovitis in early-stage osteoarthritis using a post-traumatic rat model. PLoS One 2021;16(7): e0254383. PMID: 34270585; PMCID: PMC8284605.
28. Buckwalter JA, Anderson DD, Brown TD, et al. The roles of mechanical stresses in the pathogenesis of osteoarthritis: implications for treatment of joint injuries. Cartilage 2013;4(4):286–94.
29. Fernández-Moreno M, Rego I, Carreira-Garcia V, et al. Genetics in osteoarthritis. Curr Genomics 2008;9(8): 542–7. PMID: 19516961; PMCID: PMC2694558.
30. Szala D, Kopańska M, Trojniak J, et al. The role of MicroRNAs in the pathophysiology of osteoarthritis. Int J Mol Sci 2024;25(12). https://doi.org/10.3390/ijms25126352.

31. Liu-Bryan R, Terkeltaub R. Emerging regulators of the inflammatory process in osteoarthritis. Nat Rev Rheumatol 2015;11(1):35–44.
32. Robinson WH, Lepus CM, Wang Q, et al. Low-grade inflammation as a key mediator of the pathogenesis of osteoarthritis. Nat Rev Rheumatol 2016;12(10):580–92.
33. Rahmati M, Mobasheri A, Mozafari M. Inflammatory mediators in osteoarthritis: a critical review of the state-of-the-art, current prospects, and future challenges. Bone 2016;85:81–90.
34. Uebelhoer M, Lambert C, Grisart J, et al. Interleukins, growth factors, and transcription factors are key targets for gene therapy in osteoarthritis: a scoping review. Front Med (Lausanne) 2023;10: 1148623.
35. Troeberg L, Nagase H. Proteases involved in cartilage matrix degradation in osteoarthritis. Biochim Biophys Acta 2012;1824(1):133–45.
36. Sanchez-Lopez E, Coras R, Torres A, et al. Synovial inflammation in osteoarthritis progression. Nat Rev Rheumatol 2022;18(5):258–75.
37. Sellam J, Berenbaum F. Is osteoarthritis a metabolic disease? Jt Bone Spine 2013;80(6):568–73.
38. Kluzek S, Newton JL, Arden NK. Is osteoarthritis a metabolic disorder? Br Med Bull 2015;115(1): 111–21.
39. June RK, Liu-Bryan R, Long F, et al. Emerging role of metabolic signaling in synovial joint remodeling and osteoarthritis. J Orthop Res 2016;34(12): 2048–58.
40. Mobasheri A, Rayman MP, Gualillo O, et al. The role of metabolism in the pathogenesis of osteoarthritis. Nat Rev Rheumatol 2017;13(5): 302–11.
41. Kramer WC, Hendricks KJ, Wang J. Pathogenetic mechanisms of posttraumatic osteoarthritis: opportunities for early intervention. Int J Clin Exp Med 2011;4(4):285–98.
42. Brophy RH, Fillingham YA. AAOS Clinical Practice Guideline Summary: management of Osteoarthritis of the Knee (Nonarthroplasty), 3rd edition. J Am Acad Orthop Surg 2022;30(9):e721–9.
43. Hannon CP, Delanois RE, Nandi S, et al, Management of Osteoarthritis of the Hip Work Group, Staff of the American Academy of Orthopaedic Surgeons, Management of Osteoarthritis of the Hip Work Group and Staff of the American Academy of Orthopaedic Surgeons. American Academy of Orthopaedic Surgeons Clinical Practice Guideline Summary management of osteoarthritis of the hip. J Am Acad Orthop Surg 2024;32(20): e1027–34.
44. Srivastava AK, Surgical Management of Osteoarthritis of the Knee Work Group, Staff of the American Academy of Orthopaedic Surgeons. American Academy of Orthopaedic Surgeons Clinical Practice Guideline Summary of surgical management of osteoarthritis of the knee. J Am Acad Orthop Surg 2023;31(24):1211–20.
45. Felson DT, Lawrence RC, Hochberg MC, et al. Osteoarthritis: new insights. Part 2: treatment approaches. Ann Intern Med 2000;133(9):726–37.
46. Latourte A, Kloppenburg M, Richette P. Emerging pharmaceutical therapies for osteoarthritis. Nat Rev Rheumatol 2020;16(12):673–88.
47. Robinson RL, Schnitzer TJ, Barlow S, et al. Satisfaction with medications prescribed for Osteoarthritis: a Cross-Sectional Survey of patients and their physicians in the United States. Pain Ther 2022;11(1):191–208.
48. Klem NR, Kent P, Smith A, et al. Satisfaction after total knee replacement for osteoarthritis is usually high, but what are we measuring? A systematic review. Osteoarthr Cartil Open 2020;2(1): 100032.
49. Baker CL Jr, Ferguson CM. Future treatment of osteoarthritis. Orthopedics 2005;28(2 Suppl):s227–34.
50. Evans CH, Gouze JN, Gouze E, et al. Osteoarthritis gene therapy. Gene Ther 2004;11(4):379–89.
51. Evans CH, Ghivizzani SC, Robbins PD. Orthopaedic gene therapy: Twenty-Five years on. JBJS Rev 2021;9(8).
52. Evans CH, Huard J. Gene therapy approaches to regenerating the musculoskeletal system. Nat Rev Rheumatol 2015;11(4):234–42.
53. Ginn SL, Alexander IE, Edelstein ML, et al. Gene therapy clinical trials worldwide to 2012 - an update. J Gene Med 2013;15(2):65–77.
54. Hacein-Bey-Abina S, Von Kalle C, Schmidt M, et al. LMO2-associated clonal T cell proliferation in two patients after gene therapy for SCID-X1. Science (New York, N.Y.) 2003;302(5644):415–9.
55. Raper SE, Chirmule N, Lee FS, et al. Fatal systemic inflammatory response syndrome in a ornithine transcarbamylase deficient patient following adenoviral gene transfer. Mol Genet Metabol 2003;80(1–2):148–58.
56. Rai MF, Sandell LJ. Emerging concepts in gene therapy for osteoarthritis. J Am Acad Orthop Surg 2015;23(10):e56–7.
57. Li X, Shen L, Deng Z, et al. New treatment for osteoarthritis: gene therapy. Precis Clin Med 2023;6(2):pbad014.
58. Zhu W, Niu T, Wei Z, et al. Advances in biomaterial-mediated gene therapy for articular cartilage repair. Bioengineering (Basel) 2022;9(10).
59. Chen H, Li Z, Li X, et al. Biomaterial-based gene delivery: advanced tools for enhanced cartilage regeneration. Drug Des Dev Ther 2023;17: 3605–24.
60. Evans CH, Ghivizzani SC, Robbins PD. Osteoarthritis gene therapy in 2022. Curr Opin Rheumatol 2023;35(1):37–43.

61. Evans CH, Ghivizzani SC, Robbins PD. The 2024 OREF clinical research award: progress toward a gene therapy for arthritis. J Am Acad Orthop Surg 2024;32(23):1052–60.
62. Li Y, Li B, Nagy A, et al. Application of gene therapy in osteoarthritis. Connect Tissue Res 2025; 66(5):450–7.
63. Peitso V, Ng K, Ellis R, et al. Gene therapy pipelines for osteoarthritis: current innovations, operational challenges, and future directions. Connect Tissue Res 2025;66(5):458–65.
64. Lv R, Du L, Bai L. RNF125, transcriptionally regulated by NFATC2, alleviates osteoarthritis via inhibiting the Wnt/beta-catenin signaling pathway through degrading TRIM14. Int Immunopharmacol 2023;125(Pt B):111191.
65. Kobayashi H, Chang SH, Mori D, et al. Biphasic regulation of chondrocytes by Rela through induction of anti-apoptotic and catabolic target genes. Nat Commun 2016;7:13336.
66. Ruan MZ, Erez A, Guse K, et al. Proteoglycan 4 expression protects against the development of osteoarthritis. Sci Transl Med 2013;5(176): 176ra134.
67. Kim JA, Im S, Cantley LC, et al. Suppression of Nkx3.2 by phosphatidylinositol-3-kinase signaling regulates cartilage development by modulating chondrocyte hypertrophy. Cell Signal 2015;27-(12):2389–400.
68. Park M, Yong Y, Choi SW, et al. Constitutive RelA activation mediated by Nkx3.2 controls chondrocyte viability. Nat Cell Biol 2007;9(3):287–98.
69. Yong Y, Choi SW, Choi HJ, et al. Exogenous signal-independent nuclear IkappaB kinase activation triggered by Nkx3.2 enables constitutive nuclear degradation of IkappaB-alpha in chondrocytes. Mol Cell Biol 2011;31(14):2802–16.
70. Watson-Levings RS, Palmer GD, Levings PP, et al. Gene therapy in orthopaedics: progress and challenges in pre-clinical development and translation. Front Bioeng Biotechnol 2022;10: 901317.
71. Yoon DS, Lee KM, Cho S, et al. Cellular and tissue selectivity of AAV serotypes for gene delivery to chondrocytes and cartilage. Int J Med Sci 2021;18-(15):3353–60.
72. Ruan MZ, Cerullo V, Cela R, et al. Treatment of osteoarthritis using a helper-dependent adenoviral vector retargeted to chondrocytes. Mol Ther Methods Clin Dev 2016;3:16008.
73. Li C, Samulski RJ. Engineering adeno-associated virus vectors for gene therapy. Nat Rev Genet 2020;21(4):255–72.
74. Nassini R, Chieca M, Marini M, et al. AAV vectors: an emerging strategy for chronic pain management. Trends Mol Med 2025. https://doi.org/10.1016/j.molmed.2025.08.008.
75. Nixon AJ, Grol MW, Lang HM, et al. Disease-modifying osteoarthritis treatment with Interleukin-1 receptor antagonist gene therapy in small and large animal models. Arthritis Rheumatol 2018;70(11): 1757–68.
76. Luo S, Jiang H, Li Q, et al. The intra-articular delivery of a low-dose adeno-associated Virus-IL-1 receptor antagonist vector alleviates the progress of arthritis in an osteoarthritis rat model. Pharmaceutics 2024;16(12). https://doi.org/10.3390/pharmaceutics16121518.
77. Snuggs JW, Senter RK, Whitt JP, et al. PCRX-201, a novel IL-1Ra gene therapy treatment approach for low back pain resulting from intervertebral disc degeneration. Gene Ther 2025;32(2):93–105.
78. Wang G, Evans CH, Benson JM, et al. Safety and biodistribution assessment of sc-rAAV2.5IL-1Ra administered via intra-articular injection in a mono-iodoacetate-induced osteoarthritis rat model. Mol Ther Methods Clin Dev 2016;3:15052.
79. Evans CH, Ghivizzani SC, Robbins PD. Gene delivery to joints by intra-articular injection. Hum Gene Ther 2018;29(1):2–14.
80. Watson Levings RS, Broome TA, Smith AD, et al. Gene therapy for osteoarthritis: pharmacokinetics of intra-articular self-complementary adeno-associated virus Interleukin-1 receptor antagonist delivery in an equine model. Hum Gene Ther Clin Dev 2018;29(2):90–100.
81. De la Vega RE, Sellon JL, Smith J, et al. A phase 1 clinical trial shows safe, sustained, AAV-mediated expression of IL-1Ra in the human osteoarthritic knee joint. Sci Transl Med 2025;17-(801):eadu9804.
82. Lange C, Madry H, Venkatesan JK, et al. rAAV-Mediated sox9 overexpression improves the repair of osteochondral defects in a clinically relevant large animal model over time in vivo and reduces perifocal osteoarthritic changes. Am J Sports Med 2021;49(13):3696–707.
83. Morscheid YP, Venkatesan JK, Schmitt G, et al. rAAV-Mediated human FGF-2 gene therapy enhances osteochondral repair in a clinically relevant large animal model over time in vivo. Am J Sports Med 2021;49(4):958–69.
84. Seol D, Choe HH, Zheng H, et al. Intra-articular adeno-associated virus-mediated proteoglycan 4 gene therapy for preventing posttraumatic osteoarthritis. Hum Gene Ther 2022;33(9–10):529–40.
85. Peifer C, Oláh T, Venkatesan JK, et al. Locally directed recombinant Adeno- associated virus-mediated IGF-1 gene therapy enhances osteochondral repair and counteracts early osteoarthritis in vivo. Am J Sports Med 2024;52(5):1336–49.
86. Gantenbein B, Tang S, Guerrero J, et al. Non-viral gene delivery methods for bone and joints. Front Bioeng Biotechnol 2020;8:598466.

87. Uzieliene I, Kalvaityte U, Bernotiene E, et al. Non-viral gene therapy for osteoarthritis. Front Bioeng Biotechnol 2020;8:618399.
88. Huang P, Zhao J, Wang X, et al. The application of novel drug delivery systems in the treatment of osteoarthritis. Pharmaceutics 2025;17(10). https://doi.org/10.3390/pharmaceutics17101272.
89. Fu Y, Huang Y, Wang Y, et al. Virus-inspired lipopeptide-derived nucleic acid delivery to cartilage for osteoarthritis therapy. Nat Commun 2025; 16(1):9184.
90. Yan X, Chen YR, Song YF, et al. Scaffold-based gene therapeutics for osteochondral tissue engineering. Front Pharmacol 2019;10:1534.
91. Cherian JJ, Parvizi J, Bramlet D, et al. Preliminary results of a phase II randomized study to determine the efficacy and safety of genetically engineered allogeneic human chondrocytes expressing TGF-beta1 in patients with grade 3 chronic degenerative joint disease of the knee. Osteoarthr Cartil 2015;23(12):2109–18.
92. Ha CW, Cho JJ, Elmallah RK, et al. A multicenter, single-blind, phase IIa clinical trial to evaluate the efficacy and safety of a cell-mediated gene therapy in degenerative knee arthritis patients. Hum Gene Ther Clin Dev 2015;26(2):125–30.
93. Park EH, Seo J, Lee Y, et al. TissueGene-C induces long-term analgesic effects through regulation of pain mediators and neuronal sensitization in a rat monoiodoacetate-induced model of osteoarthritis pain. Osteoarthr Cartil 2023;31(12):1567–80.
94. Shen J, Abu-Amer Y, O'Keefe JR, et al. Inflammation and epigenetic regulation in osteoarthritis. Connect Tissue Res 2017;58(1):49–63.
95. Karlsen TA, Pernas PF, Staerk J, et al. Generation of IL1β-resistant chondrocytes using CRISPR-CAS genome editing. Osteoarthr Cartil 2016;24. https://doi.org/10.1016/j.joca.2016.01.581.
96. Tanikella AS, Hardy MJ, Frahs SM, et al. Emerging gene-editing modalities for osteoarthritis. Int J Mol Sci 2020;21(17). https://doi.org/10.3390/ijms21176046.
97. Ren X, Hu B, Song M, et al. Maintenance of nucleolar homeostasis by CBX4 alleviates senescence and osteoarthritis. Cell Rep 2019;26(13):3643–56.e7.
98. Zhang J, Liu GH, Qu J, et al. Treating osteoarthritis via gene therapy with rejuvenation factors. Gene Ther 2020;27(7–8):309–11.
99. Zhang D, Cao X, Li J, et al. MiR-210 inhibits NF-kappaB signaling pathway by targeting DR6 in osteoarthritis. Sci Rep 2015;5:12775.
100. Karlsen TA, de Souza GA, Odegaard B, et al. microRNA-140 inhibits inflammation and stimulates chondrogenesis in a model of interleukin 1beta-induced osteoarthritis. Mol Ther Nucleic Acids 2016;5(10):e373.
101. Chang LH, Chuang SC, Wu SC, et al. Comparisons of miRNA profiles of exosomes derived from human iPSCs, ADSCs, and BMSCs and effects on chondrocyte function. Bone Joint Res 2025;14(8):696–712.
102. Li Z, Chen Z, Wang X, et al. Integrated analysis of miRNAs and gene expression profiles reveals potential biomarkers for osteoarthritis. Front Genet 2022;13:814645.
103. Si HB, Zeng Y, Liu SY, et al. Intra-articular injection of microRNA-140 (miRNA-140) alleviates osteoarthritis (OA) progression by modulating extracellular matrix (ECM) homeostasis in rats. Osteoarthr Cartil 2017;25(10):1698–707.
104. Shang X. Mechanosensitive miRNAs in cartilage and subchondral bone remodeling: emerging targets for osteoarthritis therapy. J Inflamm Res 2025;18:9609–25.

Glucagon-like Peptide-1 Receptor Agonist Use May Reduce Disease Activity and Progression in Osteoarthritis and Inflammatory Arthritis

Maxwell Trudeau, MD, Olivia Schaffer, BS,
Ran Schwarzkopf, MD, MSc*

KEYWORDS

• Osteoarthritis • Rheumatoid arthritis • Metabolic syndrome • Diabetes mellitus
• GLP-1 receptor agonists • Chronic inflammation • Obesity

KEY POINTS

- Osteoarthritis is increasingly recognized as metabolically driven, with obesity and metabolic syndrome promoting inflammation and degeneration.
- Glucagon-like peptide-1 (GLP-1) receptor agonists may have plausible disease-modifying effects in osteoarthritis: reduced inflammatory cytokines, oxidative stress, and matrix degradation.
- In knee osteoarthritis, randomized controlled trials show meaningful weight loss and modest improvements in pain and function for patients on GLP-1 receptor agonists.
- Limited observational and preclinical data on rheumatoid arthritis, psoriatic arthritis, and gout suggests possible reductions in disease markers after GLP-1 receptor agonist use.

INTRODUCTION

Osteoarthritis (OA) has traditionally been conceptualized as a degenerative joint disease driven primarily by aging and mechanical overload. However, growing epidemiologic and mechanistic evidence supports a central role for metabolic dysfunction in OA pathogenesis, particularly among younger individuals with obesity or type 2 diabetes mellitus (T2DM).[1] Obesity and metabolic syndrome (MetS) are associated with OA in both weight-bearing and non–weight-bearing joints, suggesting that systemic metabolic and inflammatory factors contribute to disease development beyond biomechanical stress alone.[1]

Adipose tissue functions as an active endocrine organ, producing adipokines including leptin, resistin, and lipocalin, as well as proinflammatory cytokines such as tumor necrosis factor alpha, interleukin 1, and interleukin 6. These mediators arise from both local and systemic adipose depots and may be released in response to joint trauma or chronic mechanical overuse, promoting synovial inflammation, cartilage catabolism, and progressive joint degeneration.[1] In a cohort of more than 1.7 million individuals, obesity was associated with over a threefold increased risk of knee OA compared with normal-weight individuals.[1] Metabolic dysregulation further contributes to OA through chronic hyperglycemia, oxidative stress, synovial insulin resistance, and altered lipid metabolism. Inflammatory pathways activated in MetS substantially overlap with those implicated in OA and inflammatory arthritis, positioning metabolic disease

Department of Orthopedic Surgery, NYU Langone, 301 East 17th Street, 14th Floor, New York, NY 10003, USA
* Corresponding author. Department of Orthopedic Surgery, NYU Grossman School of Medicine.
E-mail address: schwarzk@gmail.com

Orthop Clin N Am 57 (2026) 317–327
https://doi.org/10.1016/j.ocl.2026.05.004
0030-5898/26/

Abbreviation	
GLP-1	glucagon-like peptide-1
MetS	metabolic syndrome
OA	osteoarthritis
PsA	psoriatic arthritis
RCT	randomized controlled trial
T2DM	type 2 diabetes mellitus

as a shared upstream driver of musculoskeletal inflammation.[2,3]

Over the past decade, the use of glucagon-like peptide-1 receptor agonists (GLP-1 RAs) has expanded rapidly. Prescription data demonstrate marked growth in GLP-1 RA utilization across populations with T2DM, cardiovascular disease, and obesity. Semaglutide use increased from 569 users in 2019 to over 22,000 users in 2022, becoming the most frequently prescribed GLP-1 RA, particularly among overweight and obese patients.[4] Monthly growth rates exceeded 80% for multiple agents, with tirzepatide demonstrating growth rates greater than 250% (Watanabe and colleagues). In the United States, the proportion of adults with T2DM treated with GLP-1 RAs increased from 4.3% in 2016 to 19.4% in 2022, with inflation-adjusted expenditures reaching 33.9 billion dollars annually.[5] Importantly, GLP-1 RA initiation among overweight or obese individuals without diabetes increased more than 700% between 2019 and 2023.[6] This widespread adoption raises important questions regarding the downstream musculoskeletal and perioperative effects of these therapies.

GLP-1 is an incretin hormone secreted by the intestine in response to nutrient ingestion. Activation of the GLP-1 receptor enhances glucose-dependent insulin secretion, suppresses glucagon release, delays gastric emptying, and reduces appetite, collectively improving glycemic control and promoting weight loss.[7] Beyond metabolic regulation, GLP-1 RAs exert pleiotropic effects relevant to joint disease. In OA, chondrocytes and synovial cells respond to inflammatory cytokines, mechanical stress, and extracellular matrix disruption by activating catabolic and apoptotic pathways. Incretin mimetics that bind the GLP-1 receptor demonstrate immunomodulatory, anti-inflammatory, and cytoprotective effects that may counteract these processes.[2] In rheumatic diseases including rheumatoid arthritis and psoriatic arthritis (PsA), GLP-1 RAs modulate inflammatory signaling, oxidative stress, and immune cell activation, suggesting a potentially beneficial disease-modifying effect across inflammatory arthritis phenotypes.[8]

Arthritis phenotypes beyond OA are consistently associated with greater surgical complexity and worse outcomes following total joint arthroplasty, largely due to higher baseline systemic inflammation and metabolic comorbidity. Patients with rheumatoid arthritis and PsA experience significantly increased perioperative risk, including an approximately 50% higher rate of periprosthetic joint infection compared with OA, a risk further amplified by the high prevalence of obesity and its independent associations with infection, thromboembolism, and mechanical complications.[9–12] Similarly, gout affects approximately 4% to 6% of arthroplasty patients and is associated with higher rates of wound complications, infection, and revision surgery, with risk escalating markedly when gout coexists with obesity or MetS.[13–16] Across these inflammatory and crystal arthropathies, perioperative management is complicated by immunosuppressive therapies, frequent disease flares, technical challenges related to body habitus, and the need for broader preoperative evaluation due to polyarticular and axial involvement, with current guidelines emphasizing infection risk mitigation even at the expense of postoperative flares.[17,18] Non-OA arthritis populations are not only more likely to require surgery but are also inherently harder to manage surgically, underscoring that effective control of systemic inflammation and metabolic dysfunction may be critical not only to delay arthroplasty but also to render these patients safer and more manageable surgical candidates.

The purpose of this review is to synthesize and critically evaluate the current preclinical, observational, and clinical evidence regarding the role of GLP-1 RAs in the management of arthritis, with particular emphasis on OA, gouty arthritis, and inflammatory arthritis phenotypes relevant to orthopedic practice. By contextualizing the metabolic, inflammatory, and musculoskeletal effects of GLP-1 RAs alongside emerging clinical data, this review aims to provide orthopedic surgeons with an evidence-based framework to inform patient counseling and perioperative risk assessment. Given the rapid expansion of GLP-1 RA use among patients with obesity, MetS, and T2DM, an understanding of their potential benefits in arthritis management is increasingly essential for contemporary orthopedic practice.

CURRENT EVIDENCE

Preclinical Evidence

The GLP-1 receptor is expressed in articular cartilage, synovium, meniscal tissue, and subchondral bone in both healthy and diseased models. In degenerative cartilage, receptor expression is reduced relative to healthy tissue, and advanced glycation end products further suppress receptor expression in chondrocytes exposed to a diabetic milieu. In rodent models of monosodium iodoacetate–induced OA, similar downregulation of receptor expression occurs, and treatment with the GLP-1 RA liraglutide increases receptor expression relative to untreated controls.[19,20]

Preclinical functional studies demonstrate that GLP-1 RAs exert analgesic and anti-inflammatory effects in injured joint environments. In a murine model of knee OA, intra-articular administration of liraglutide produced rapid and sustained increases in mechanical pain thresholds relative to baseline. In head-to-head comparisons with dexamethasone, liraglutide matched or exceeded corticosteroid treatment in reducing pain over time and attenuated histologic measures of synovitis. These effects occurred independently of weight change in some experimental designs. Additional studies demonstrated reductions in tumor necrosis factor alpha, interleukin 1, and interleukin 6 at both gene and protein levels in chondrocytes and macrophages following GLP-1 RA treatment.[21–24]

Oxidative stress and extracellular matrix degradation are central components of OA pathogenesis that may be modulated by GLP-1 RA therapy. *In vitro* studies demonstrate that GLP-1 RAs reduce reactive oxygen species production and restore antioxidant capacity in chondrocytes exposed to advanced glycation end products or inflammatory cytokines. In models of catabolic imbalance, these agents downregulate enzymes responsible for cartilage matrix degradation (such as matrix metalloproteinases) while preserving type II collagen and aggrecan content. GLP-1 RAs also modulate apoptosis and promote autophagy in chondrocytes, reducing activation of pro-apoptotic signaling pathways and enhancing expression of autophagy markers (**Fig. 1**A). These findings are supported by evidence demonstrating restoration of mitochondrial function under conditions of metabolic stress.[19,23,24]

Preclinical evidence in inflammatory arthritis demonstrates that GLP-1 RAs exert anti-inflammatory and immunomodulatory effects through multiple mechanisms that appear partially independent of weight loss. In rheumatoid arthritis models, GLP-1 RAs inhibit nuclear factor kappa B signaling, reduce proinflammatory cytokines including tumor necrosis factor, interleukin 6, and interleukin 17, and modulate macrophage activity (see **Fig. 1**B). Additional studies demonstrate suppression of the NLRP3 inflammasome and c-Jun N-terminal kinase pathways, which have been implicated in the pathogenesis of rheumatic diseases. In PsA models, GLP-1 RAs reduce tumor necrosis factor, interleukin 6, and interleukin 17, cytokines central to both cutaneous and articular disease manifestations.[25] Collectively, these findings highlight tissue-specific but convergent anti-inflammatory effects of GLP-1 RAs across inflammatory arthritis phenotypes.[26] The mechanism by which GLP-1 RAs modify disease activity in gout is likely through increased renal uric acid excretion mediated by inhibition of the sodium-hydrogen exchanger type 3 in the proximal tubule,[27] although the exact mechanism has not been elucidated by preclinical studies.

Observational Studies

Prospective and retrospective observational studies evaluating GLP-1 RA exposure in OA and inflammatory arthritis provide mixed but informative signals regarding symptomatic relief, structural outcomes, and disease incidence. In knee OA, Zhu and colleagues (2023) performed a large multicenter prospective cohort study in China enrolling patients with concomitant knee OA and T2DM (Kellgren–Lawrence grades 1–3).[28] Over a mean follow-up of approximately 5 to 8 years, 233 GLP-1 RA users were compared with 1574 nonusers, with broadly similar background antidiabetic therapy between groups. GLP-1 RA use was associated with lower rates of knee surgery, reduced use of analgesics and intra-articular interventions, and significantly improved WOMAC scores. Notably, imaging analyses demonstrated relative preservation of medial femorotibial cartilage thickness among GLP-1 RA users, raising the possibility of structural modification rather than purely symptomatic benefit.

Shorter-term symptomatic effects have been reported in smaller observational cohorts. Samajdar and colleagues (2024) conducted a single-arm, record-based study in India including 98 older adults with knee OA and T2DM who remained symptomatic despite conventional therapy.[29] Addition of dulaglutide to existing regimens over 6 months was associated with improvements in pain scores, reduced nonsteroidal anti-inflammatory drug use, and decreases in body weight and body mass index, alongside expected

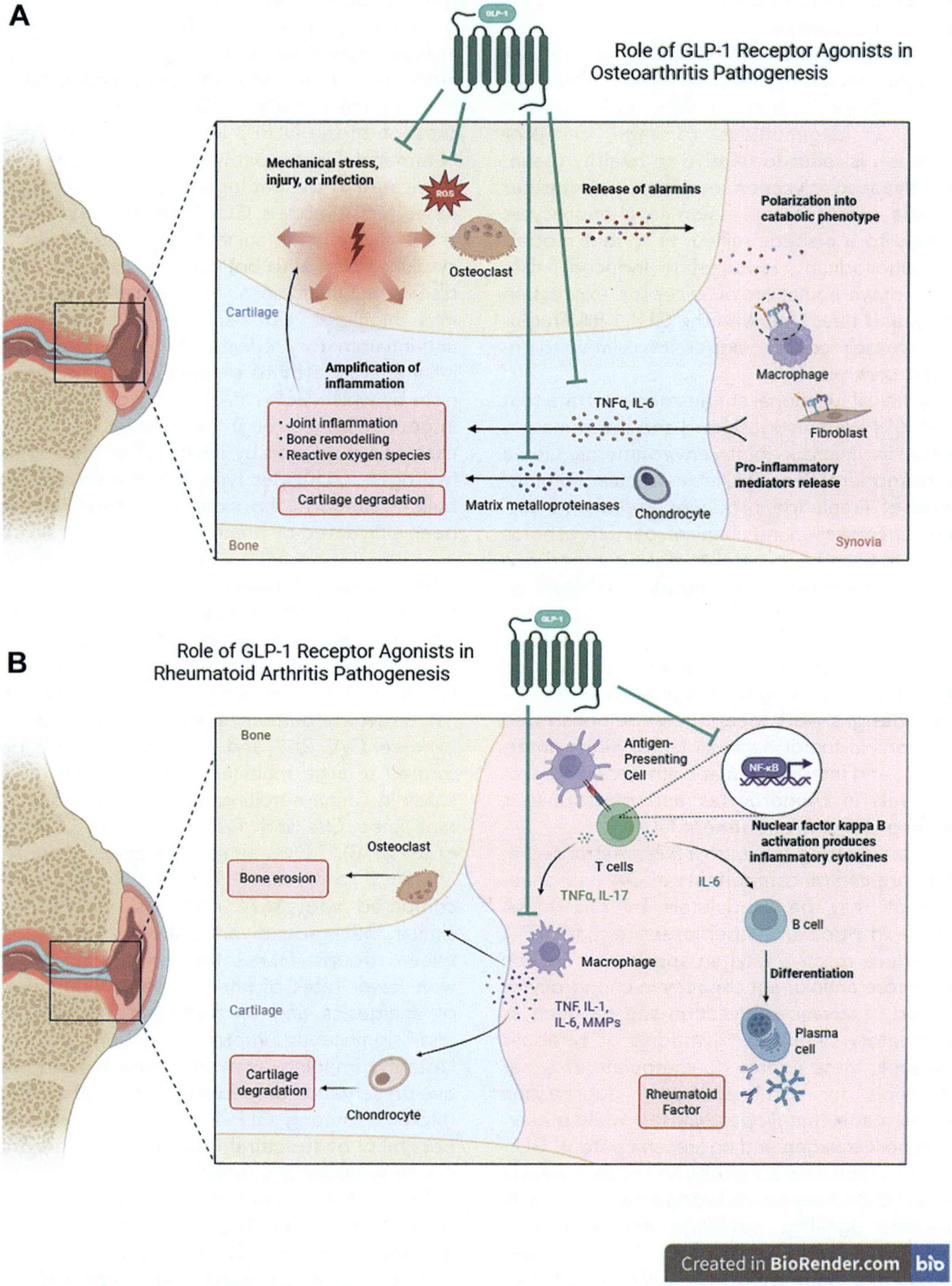

Fig. 1. Proposed mechanisms for GLP-1 RA as a disease modifier in OA and rheumatoid arthritis. IL, interleukin; MMP, matrix metalloproteinase; TNFα, tumor necrosis factor alpha. (Created in BioRender. Schaffer, O. (2026). https://BioRender.com/0y8tp9y.)

improvements in glycemic control. Although the absence of a comparator group precludes causal inference, the consistent temporal relationship between GLP-1 RA initiation and symptom improvement supports a potential functional benefit in symptomatic knee OA.

In contrast, some retrospective database analyses have yielded neutral findings. Lavu and colleagues (2024) evaluated knee OA development and total knee arthroplasty rates in US cohorts stratified by obesity and T2DM status, excluding patients with pre-existing hip or knee OA and requiring at least 5 years of follow-up.[30] Among obese patients with T2DM, more than 15,000 matched individuals per group showed no significant differences in knee OA diagnosis or arthroplasty rates between GLP-1 RA users and nonusers, despite improvements in metabolic parameters. Similar results were observed in obese nondiabetic and nonobese diabetic cohorts. These findings suggest that while GLP-1 RAs reliably improve metabolic health, their impact on OA incidence or progression to surgical intervention may be limited within the observed time frames.

Evidence from inflammatory arthritis cohorts provides additional mechanistic context. Kellner and colleagues reported a retrospective chart review of patients with rheumatoid arthritis and elevated body mass index treated with semaglutide or tirzepatide, demonstrating reductions in disease activity scores, pain, inflammatory markers, and cardiometabolic risk factors compared with controls, though treatment discontinuation was common due to gastrointestinal adverse effects. Smaller prospective observational studies using liraglutide in rheumatoid arthritis and PsA similarly reported improvements in DAS-28 scores, swollen joint counts, and inflammatory biomarkers, with correlations between weight loss and disease activity reduction.[31,32] While limited by small sample sizes and nonrandomized designs, these studies suggest potential anti-inflammatory or immunomodulatory effects of GLP-1 RAs beyond weight reduction alone.

Finally, several observational studies have examined biochemical pathways relevant to crystal arthropathy, reporting modest but consistent reductions in serum uric acid with GLP-1 RA therapy.[33–37] However, none of these studies measured the association between GLP-1 RA utilization and gout flare frequency or severity relevant to orthopedic practice.

Randomized Clinical Trials

Several randomized controlled trials (RCTs) have evaluated GLP-1 RA therapy in patients with knee OA and overweight or obesity, with heterogeneity in study design, eligibility criteria, intervention duration, and primary endpoints. Collectively, these trials provide controlled evidence regarding weight loss, pain reduction, and functional outcomes, while offering limited insight into structural disease modification.

Bartholdy and colleagues conducted a randomized, placebo-controlled trial in Denmark enrolling adults aged 18 to 74 years with radiographically confirmed knee OA and overweight or obesity.[38] Participants first completed an intensive dietary intervention to achieve at least 5% weight loss before randomization. Those assigned to liraglutide received dose escalation from 0.6 mg daily to a target dose of 3.0 mg daily and were followed for 52 weeks. Compared with placebo, liraglutide resulted in significantly greater weight loss and improvements in functional outcomes measured by the Knee Injury and Osteoarthritis Outcome Score, along with increased physical activity. These findings support additive metabolic and functional benefits of GLP-1 RA therapy following weight loss induction.

Bliddal and colleagues subsequently evaluated once-weekly semaglutide in a double-blind RCT enrolling adults with obesity (body mass index $\geq$30) and symptomatic knee OA, defined by baseline Western Ontario and McMaster Universities Osteoarthritis Index (WOMAC) pain scores $\geq$40 on a 0 to 100 scale.[39] Semaglutide was escalated from 0.24 mg to a target dose of 2.4 mg by week 16, with a total treatment duration of 68 weeks. Semaglutide-treated patients experienced significantly greater reductions in body weight and WOMAC pain scores compared with placebo, along with improvements in health-related quality of life assessed by the Short Form-36 (SF-36). Gastrointestinal adverse events were more common in the semaglutide arm, consistent with the known safety profile of GLP-1 RAs.

Gudbergsen and colleagues reported a related Danish RCT focusing on the maintenance of weight loss and symptom control.[40] After an 8-week dietary induction achieving at least 5% weight loss, participants with knee OA were randomized to liraglutide or placebo for 52 weeks. Liraglutide therapy sustained weight reduction and was associated with modest improvements in validated pain measures, including knee injury and osteoarthrits outcome scores (KOOS) pain, intermittent and constant osteoarthritis pain (ICOAP), and WOMAC scores. However, not all pain endpoints reached statistical significance, suggesting that the symptomatic benefits of liraglutide in knee OA may be largely mediated through weight loss rather than a direct analgesic or disease-modifying effect.

RCTs examining the impact of GLP-1 RAs on serum uric acid have demonstrated heterogeneous and generally modest effects. In patients with T2DM, several placebo- or standard-of-care–controlled trials showed no significant between-group differences in serum uric acid, including studies of exenatide (Dutour, 2016), dulaglutide (Kuchay, 2020), and liraglutide (Liakos, 2019).[41–43] In contrast, select trials reported significant urate reductions, including a Chinese RCT of IB1362 in patients with obesity and hyperphagia (Ji, 2021) and a Danish trial of liraglutide in T2DM (Zobbe, 2020).[44,45] Head-to-head trials suggest that GLP-1 RAs may be less effective for urate lowering than alternative glucose-lowering agents, with exenatide inferior to insulin glargine plus metformin (Muskiet, 2019) and liraglutide producing smaller reductions than empagliflozin (Nakaguchi, 2020).[46,47] A meta-analysis identified a statistically significant but modest overall reduction in serum uric acid with GLP-1 RA therapy, with a smaller magnitude of effect than that observed with insulin, metformin, or SGLT2 inhibitors.[48] Taken together, these findings suggest that GLP-1 RAs may confer ancillary urate-lowering effects but are unlikely to serve as primary therapies for gouty arthritis.

No completed RCTs have evaluated GLP-1 RAs in rheumatoid arthritis or PsA. However, multiple trials are ongoing or planned across OA and inflammatory rheumatic diseases. In systemic sclerosis, a randomized trial in China (NCT06149260) is evaluating subcutaneous semaglutide with improvement in modified Rodnan skin score at 24 weeks as the primary endpoint. The TOGETHER-PsA trial (NCT06588296) is a Phase 3b open-label study comparing ixekizumab alone versus ixekizumab combined with tirzepatide in patients with PsA. In knee OA, the STOP KNEE-OA trial (NCT06191848) is assessing tirzepatide in obese patients awaiting knee replacement, with arthroplasty rates within 72 weeks as the primary outcome. The NPO-OOPS-TKR study (NCT06807970) in Hong Kong is designed to optimize perioperative obesity management using semaglutide, with pain intensity as the primary endpoint, though recruitment has not yet begun. Together, these trials reflect growing international interest in defining the role of GLP-1 RAs across musculoskeletal and rheumatic diseases, with endpoints spanning symptomatic improvement, metabolic optimization, and surgical avoidance.

DISCUSSION

Across preclinical, observational, and randomized clinical studies, GLP-1 RAs demonstrate biologically plausible and clinically relevant effects that intersect with arthritis pathophysiology and orthopedic outcomes (**Table 1**). Preclinical models consistently show that GLP-1 RAs reduce synovial inflammation, oxidative stress, chondrocyte apoptosis, and cartilage matrix degradation while modulating cytokines central to OA and inflammatory arthritis, including tumor necrosis factor, interleukin 1, interleukin 6, and interleukin 17.[8,19,20,22] These effects appear at least partially independent of weight loss, in experimental systems, supporting a potential direct joint-level mechanism.

Clinical evidence in OA is strongest for symptomatic improvement and weight-mediated benefit. Randomized trials in knee OA consistently demonstrate that GLP-1 RA therapy results in significant weight loss and modest but clinically meaningful improvements in pain and function, as measured by WOMAC, KOOS, ICOAP, and SF-36 scores.[38–40] Trials incorporating dietary weight loss induction suggest that GLP-1 RAs may help sustain weight reduction and associated symptom improvement rather than exerting a dominant independent analgesic effect. Observational data from Zhu and colleagues (2023) further suggest potential structural and surgical benefits, including cartilage preservation and reduced knee surgery rates,[28] though these findings are not uniformly replicated in large retrospective datasets.[30]

Evidence in inflammatory arthritis remains limited but suggestive. Observational studies in rheumatoid arthritis and PsA demonstrate reductions in disease activity scores, inflammatory markers, and pain with GLP-1 RA exposure, particularly among patients with obesity.[49] Preclinical data support immunomodulatory effects across multiple inflammatory pathways relevant to rheumatic disease.[50] However, no completed randomized trials have yet evaluated GLP-1 RAs as adjunctive therapies in rheumatoid arthritis or PsA.

With respect to gouty arthritis, randomized trials demonstrate heterogeneous and generally modest effects of GLP-1 RAs on serum uric acid. While some placebo-controlled studies show statistically significant urate reductions,[44,45] others show no difference compared with control or inferiority to insulin, metformin, or SGLT2 inhibitors.[41–43,46,47] A meta-analysis supports a small overall reduction in serum uric acid that may translate into fewer gout flares, but the magnitude of effect is unlikely to improve upon standard urate-lowering therapy.[48]

Limitations

The current evidence base is limited by substantial heterogeneity in study design, patient populations, outcome measures, and duration of follow-up. Most OA trials focus exclusively on the knee, limiting generalizability to hip OA or other joints commonly treated by orthopedic

Table 1
Evidence summary for disease-modifying activity of GLP-1 RAs in arthritis

Disease	Strength of Preclinical Evidence	Strength of Observational Evidence	Strength of Randomized Trial Evidence	Evidence Strength	Quality of Evidence
Osteoarthritis	Strong: Consistent models show reduced inflammation, cartilage degradation, apoptosis, and oxidative stress	Moderate: Prospective cohorts show symptom improvement; large databases show mixed effects.	Moderate: Randomized control trials demonstrate weight loss with modest, consistent improvements in pain and function	Moderate	Moderate
Rheumatoid arthritis/PsA	Strong: Robust anti-inflammatory and immunomodulatory effects across multiple validated inflammatory arthritis models	Weak: Small, nonrandomized studies suggest improved disease activity, confounded by weight loss	Weak: No completed randomized trials evaluating clinical efficacy in inflammatory arthritis.	Low	Low
Gout	Weak: Increased renal urate excretion, exact mechanism unknown.	Moderate: Consistent modest serum urate reductions; limited data on clinical gout outcomes or effects on joints.	Weak: Modest urate lowering effects, inferior to standard urate-lowering therapies, no joint-specific data.	Moderate	Moderate

surgeons. Structural endpoints are inconsistently assessed, and few studies are powered to detect differences in surgical outcomes such as arthroplasty rates. In observational studies, confounding by indication and baseline disease severity remains difficult to fully address, particularly in metabolically complex populations.

In inflammatory arthritis, available data are largely observational, involve small sample sizes, and often emphasize systemic or laboratory outcomes rather than joint-specific or surgical endpoints. Across all arthritis phenotypes, it remains challenging to disentangle the effects of weight loss from direct anti-inflammatory or chondroprotective mechanisms. Long-term safety, durability of musculoskeletal benefit, and effects on disease progression remain incompletely characterized.

Clinical Relevance

For orthopedic surgeons, the primary relevance of GLP-1 RAs lies in their role as adjunctive therapies that address upstream metabolic drivers of arthritis severity and surgical risk. In OA, GLP-1 RAs may be considered as part of a comprehensive nonoperative management strategy for patients with obesity or T2DM, with evidence supporting improvements in pain, function, and weight that may delay surgical intervention in selected patients. In inflammatory arthritis, GLP-1 RAs may complement disease-modifying therapy by improving metabolic health and potentially attenuating inflammatory burden, though they should not be viewed as substitutes for rheumatologic treatment. For patients with gout or hyperuricemia, GLP-1 RAs may offer modest ancillary urate-lowering effects and metabolic optimization but are unlikely to replace established gout therapies. Across all populations, these agents may improve patient readiness for surgery by reducing obesity-related risk factors that are strongly associated with complications, revision surgery, and prolonged recovery.

GLP-1 RAs are associated with gastrointestinal adverse effects, including nausea, vomiting, and delayed gastric emptying, which raise specific perioperative concerns related to aspiration risk. Regulatory warnings highlight the potential for retained gastric contents despite standard fasting protocols, prompting recommendations for individualized perioperative management rather than universal medication cessation.[51] While increased gastric residual volumes have been observed, large clinical datasets suggest that the absolute risk of aspiration events remains low and comparable to historical baselines.[52]

Emerging surgical outcome data suggest potential benefits of continued GLP-1 RA therapy in the perioperative period. Observational analyses demonstrate associations with reduced readmission rates, wound complications, and hematoma formation without increased infection or bleeding risk.[53] In the context of total joint arthroplasty, recent data suggest lower periprosthetic joint infection rates, reduced readmissions, and fewer revision surgeries among GLP-1 RA users, including both diabetic and nondiabetic patients.[54–56] While causality cannot be established, these findings suggest that the metabolic and anti-inflammatory benefits of GLP-1 RAs may outweigh perioperative risks in appropriately selected patients.

SUMMARY

GLP-1 RAs exhibit biologically plausible and clinically promising effects across OA, inflammatory arthritis, and gout, particularly among patients with obesity or metabolic dysfunction. Current evidence supports their role in symptom improvement, metabolic optimization, and surgical risk reduction rather than definitive disease modification. For orthopedic surgeons, GLP-1 RAs should be viewed as adjunctive tools within multidisciplinary care models that address the metabolic contributors to arthritis and perioperative risk. Ongoing randomized trials will be essential to clarify their long-term impact on structural progression and surgical avoidance.

CLINICS CARE POINTS

- Glucagon-like peptide-1 (GLP-1) receptor agonists may be a useful adjunct in nonoperative osteoarthritis management for patients with obesity or type 2 diabetes.
- Perioperative management may benefit from interdisciplinary planning between surgery and anesthesia given gastrointestinal effects and aspiration-related considerations.
- Counseling should emphasize appropriate scope of benefit: GLP-1 receptor agonists may support metabolic optimization and potentially reduce inflammatory burden, but they are not substitutes for disease-modifying therapy in inflammatory arthritis or urate-lowering therapy in gout.

DISCLOSURE

The authors have nothing to disclose.

REFERENCES

1. Wei G, Lu K, Umar M, et al. Risk of metabolic abnormalities in osteoarthritis: a new perspective to understand its pathological mechanisms. Bone Res 2023;11(1):63.
2. Meurot C, Jacques C, Martin C, et al. Targeting the GLP-1/GLP-1R axis to treat osteoarthritis: a new opportunity? J Orthop Transl 2022;32:121–9.
3. Li J, Zhang B, Liu WX, et al. Metformin limits osteoarthritis development and progression through activation of AMPK signalling. Ann Rheum Dis 2020;79(5):635–45.
4. Watanabe JH, Kwon J, Nan B, et al. Trends in glucagon-like peptide 1 receptor agonist use, 2014 to 2022. J Am Pharm Assoc 2024;64(1):133–8.
5. Hegland TA, Fang Z, Bucher K. GLP-1 medication use for type 2 diabetes has soared. JAMA 2024; 332(12):952.
6. Mahase E. GLP-1 agonists: US sees 700% increase over four years in number of patients without diabetes starting treatment. BMJ 2024;386:q1645.
7. Andersen A, Lund A, Knop FK, et al. Glucagon-like peptide 1 in health and disease. Nat Rev Endocrinol 2018;14(7):390–403.
8. Bilgin E, Venerito V, Bogdanos DP. Glucagon-like peptide-1 (GLP-1) receptor agonists in rheumatology: a review of current evidence and future directions. Autoimmun Rev 2025;24(9):103864.
9. Goodman SM, Springer BD, Chen AF, et al. 2022 American college of rheumatology/American Association of Hip and Knee Surgeons Guideline for the perioperative management of antirheumatic medication in patients with rheumatic diseases undergoing elective total hip or total knee arthroplasty. Arthritis Care Res 2022;74(9):1399–408.
10. Charalambous A, Pincus D, High S, et al. Association of surgical experience with risk of complication in total hip arthroplasty among patients with severe obesity. JAMA Netw Open 2021;4(9):e2123478.
11. Van Den Bosch F, Coates L. Clinical management of psoriatic arthritis. Lancet 2018;391(10136): 2285–94.
12. Hannon CP, Goodman SM, Austin MS, et al. 2023 American college of rheumatology and American Association of hip and Knee Surgeons Clinical Practice Guideline for the optimal timing of elective hip or knee arthroplasty for patients with symptomatic Moderate-to-Severe osteoarthritis or advanced symptomatic osteonecrosis with secondary arthritis for whom nonoperative therapy is ineffective. Arthritis Care Res 2023;75(11):2227–38.
13. Rosas S, Zuskov A, Luo TD, et al. Gout as a predictor of total knee arthroplasty outcomes and costs. J Knee Surg 2022;35(04):362–6.
14. Cole MW, Collins LK, Wilder JH, et al. The effects of gout following total knee arthroplasty: a retrospective analysis. J Arthroplast 2023;38(8): 1499–503.
15. Kuo CF, Chou IJ, See LC, et al. Urate-lowering treatment and risk of total joint replacement in patients with gout. Rheumatology 2018;57(12):2129–39.
16. Thottam GE, Krasnokutsky S, Pillinger MH. Gout and metabolic syndrome: a tangled web. Curr Rheumatol Rep 2017;19(10):60.
17. Goodman SM. Rheumatoid arthritis: perioperative management of biologics and DMARDs. Semin Arthritis Rheum 2015;44(6):627–32.
18. Goodman SM, Figgie M. Lower extremity arthroplasty in patients with inflammatory arthritis: preoperative and perioperative management. J Am Acad Orthop Surg 2013;21(6):355–63.
19. Chen J, Xie JJ, Shi KS, et al. Glucagon-like peptide-1 receptor regulates endoplasmic reticulum stress-induced apoptosis and the associated inflammatory response in chondrocytes and the progression of osteoarthritis in rat. Cell Death Dis 2018;9(2):212.
20. Meurot C, Martin C, Sudre L, et al. Liraglutide, a glucagon-like peptide 1 receptor agonist, exerts analgesic, anti-inflammatory and anti-degradative actions in osteoarthritis. Sci Rep 2022;12(1):1567.
21. Mei J, Sun J, Wu J, et al. Liraglutide suppresses TNF-α-induced degradation of extracellular matrix in human chondrocytes: a therapeutic implication in osteoarthritis. Am J Transl Res 2019;11(8):4800–8.
22. Tong C, Liang H, Liu X, et al. The protective effects of exenatide against AGEs-induced articular matrix degradation in human primary chondrocytes. Am J Transl Res 2019;11(4):2081–9.
23. Zhang X, Jiang J, Xu J, et al. Liraglutide, a glucagon-like peptide-1 receptor agonist, ameliorates inflammation and apoptosis via inhibition of receptor for advanced glycation end products signaling in AGEs induced chondrocytes. BMC Musculoskelet Disord 2024;25(1):601.
24. Li H, Chen J, Li B, et al. The protective effects of dulaglutide against advanced glycation end products (AGEs)-induced degradation of type - collagen and aggrecan in human SW1353 chondrocytes. Chem Biol Interact 2020;322:108968.
25. Buonanno S, Gaggiano C, Terribili R, et al. The potential role of GLP-1 receptor agonists in the management of psoriatic disease: a scoping review. Inflamm Res 2025;74(1):167.
26. Bendotti G, Montefusco L, Lunati ME, et al. The anti-inflammatory and immunological properties of GLP-1 receptor agonists. Pharmacol Res 2022; 182:106320.
27. Tonneijck L, Muskiet MHA, Smits MM, et al. Postprandial renal haemodynamic effect of lixisenatide vs once-daily insulin-glulisine in patients with type 2 diabetes on insulin-glargine: an 8-week, randomised, open-label trial. Diabetes Obes Metab 2017;19(12):1669–80.

28. Zhu H, Zhou L, Wang Q, et al. Glucagon-like peptide-1 receptor agonists as a disease-modifying therapy for knee osteoarthritis mediated by weight loss: findings from the Shanghai Osteoarthritis Cohort. Ann Rheum Dis 2023;82(9):1218–26.
29. Samajdar SS, Bhaduri G, Ghoshal PK, et al. Dual effects of dulaglutide on glycemic control and knee osteoarthritis pain in elderly patients with Type 2 diabetes. Pain Manag 2024;14(7):365–73.
30. Lavu MS, Porto JR, Hecht CJ, et al. The five-year incidence of progression to osteoarthritis and total joint arthroplasty in patients prescribed glucagon-like peptide 1 receptor agonists. J Arthroplast 2024;39(10):2433–9.e1.
31. Sullivan C, Gaoatswe G, Gibney J, et al. Treatment with the glucagon-like peptide-1 analogue liraglutide is associated with amelioration of disease activity in a prospective cohort study of patients with inflammatory arthritis. In: American College of rheumatology. 2013. Available at: https://acrabstracts.org/abstract/treatment-with-the-glucagon-like-peptide-1-analogue-liraglutide-is-associated-with-amelioration-of-disease-activity-in-a-prospective-cohort-study-of-patients-with-inflammatory-arthritis/. Accessed January 27, 2026 2013.
32. Nicolau J, Nadal A, Ros I, et al. Effects of liraglutide among patients with psoriatic arthritis and obesity. Reumatol Clínica Engl Ed 2025;21(1):501809.
33. Moreno-Pérez O, Tejera-Muñoz A, Carreño-Valdivia R, et al. Impact of oral semaglutide on serum urate levels in people with type 2 diabetes: a retrospective real-world analysis (URISEMA study). Semin Arthritis Rheum 2025;74:152807.
34. Chou C, Chuang S. Evaluation of the efficacy of low-dose liraglutide in weight control among Taiwanese non-diabetes patients. J Diabetes Investig 2020;11(6):1524–31.
35. Hiramatsu T, Asano Y, Mabuchi M, et al. Liraglutide relieves cardiac dilated function than DPP -4 inhibitors. Eur J Clin Invest 2018;48(10):e13007.
36. Hiramatsu T, Ito H, Okumura S, et al. Impact of glucagon like peptide-1 receptor agonist and sodium glucose cotransporter 2 inhibitors on type 2 diabetes patients with renal impairment. Diab Vasc Dis Res 2020;17(6):1479164120971220.
37. Adropin TK. Potential link in cardiovascular protection for obese male type 2 diabetes mellitus patients treated with liraglutide. Acta Clin Croat 2020;59(Suppl 2):S133–4.
38. Bartholdy C, Overgaard A, Gudbergsen H, et al. Changes in physical activity during a one-year weight loss trial with liraglutide vs placebo in participants with knee osteoarthritis: secondary analyses of a randomised controlled trial. Osteoarthr Cartil Open 2022;4(2):100255.
39. Bliddal H, Bays H, Czernichow S, et al. Once-weekly semaglutide in persons with obesity and knee osteoarthritis. N Engl J Med 2024;391(17):1573–83.
40. Gudbergsen H, Overgaard A, Henriksen M, et al. Liraglutide after diet-induced weight loss for pain and weight control in knee osteoarthritis: a randomized controlled trial. Am J Clin Nutr 2021;113(2):314–23.
41. Dutour A, Abdesselam I, Ancel P, et al. Exenatide decreases liver fat content and epicardial adipose tissue in patients with obesity and type 2 diabetes: a prospective randomized clinical trial using magnetic resonance imaging and spectroscopy. Diabetes Obes Metab 2016;18(9):882–91.
42. Kuchay MS, Krishan S, Mishra SK, et al. Effect of dulaglutide on liver fat in patients with type 2 diabetes and NAFLD: randomised controlled trial (D-LIFT trial). Diabetologia 2020;63(11):2434–45.
43. Liakos A, Lambadiari V, Bargiota A, et al. Effect of liraglutide on ambulatory blood pressure in patients with hypertension and type 2 diabetes: a randomized, double-blind, placebo-controlled trial. Diabetes Obes Metab 2019;21(3):517–24.
44. Ji L, Jiang H, An P, et al. IBI362 (LY3305677), a weekly-dose GLP-1 and glucagon receptor dual agonist, in Chinese adults with overweight or obesity: a randomised, placebo-controlled, multiple ascending dose phase 1b study. EClinicalMedicine 2021;39:101088.
45. Zobbe K, Nielsen SM, Christensen R, et al. OP0172 effect of weight loss and liraglutide on serum urate levels among obese knee osteoarthritis patients: secondary analysis of a randomised controlled trial. Ann Rheum Dis 2020;79:107–8.
46. Muskiet MHA, Bunck MC, Heine RJ, et al. Exenatide twice-daily does not affect renal function or albuminuria compared to titrated insulin glargine in patients with type 2 diabetes mellitus: a post-hoc analysis of a 52-week randomised trial. Diabetes Res Clin Pract 2019;153:14–22.
47. Nakaguchi H, Kondo Y, Kyohara M, et al. Effects of liraglutide and empagliflozin added to insulin therapy in patients with type 2 diabetes: a randomized controlled study. J Diabetes Investig 2020;11(6):1542–50.
48. Najafi S, Bahrami M, Butler AE, et al. The effect of glucagon-like peptide-1 receptor agonists on serum uric acid concentration: a systematic review and meta-analysis. Br J Clin Pharmacol 2022;88(8):3627–37.
49. Kellner DA, Dente E, Tran V, et al. Effect of glucagon-like peptide 1 receptor agonists on patients with rheumatoid arthritis. ACR Open Rheumatol 2025;7(9):e70103.
50. Du X, Zhang H, Zhang W, et al. The protective effects of lixisenatide against inflammatory response in human rheumatoid arthritis fibroblast-like synoviocytes. Int Immunopharmacol 2019;75:105732.

51. ElSayed NA, McCoy RG, Aleppo G, et al, American Diabetes Association Professional Practice Committee. 16. Diabetes care in the hospital: standards of care in diabetes—2025. Diabetes Care 2025;48(Supplement_1):S321–34.
52. Moiz A, Filion KB, Tsoukas MA, et al. The expanding role of GLP-1 receptor agonists: a narrative review of current evidence and future directions. eClinicalMedicine 2025;86:103363.
53. Aschen SZ, Zhang A, O'Connell GM, et al. Association of perioperative glucagon-like peptide-1 receptor agonist use and postoperative outcomes. Ann Surg 2025;281(4):600–7.
54. Lee V, Durkee SM, Ponce BA, et al. Impact of glucagon-like peptide-1 receptor agonists on postoperative outcomes in arthroplasty: a systematic review. J Arthroplast 2025;40(12):3073–9.
55. Levidy MF, Vatsia S, Gohel N, et al. The effects of glucagon-like peptide-1 agonist therapy on risk of infection, fracture, and early revision in primary total joint arthroplasty. J Am Acad Orthop Surg 2025;33(21):1213–8.
56. Verhey JT, Austin RP, Tarabichi S, et al. GLP-1 agonists for weight loss: do they increase complications in non-diabetic patients undergoing primary total hip arthroplasty? J Arthroplast 2025;40(8):S101–7.

Trauma

Technological Advances in Synthetic Electrospun Materials for Soft-tissue Reconstruction following Musculoskeletal Trauma: A Review

Christopher Cosgrove, MD[a,*], Emily Sallade, BS, CCRC[b]

KEYWORDS

- Synthetic matrix • Orthopedic trauma • Reconstructive surgery • Infection • Open fracture
- Soft-tissue reinforcement • Review • Polymer matrix

KEY POINTS

- Synthetic electrospun fiber materials (SEFM) offers a versatile synthetic alternative for both topical wound healing and subdermal soft-tissue reinforcement in orthopedic trauma.
- Clinical evidence shows high closure rates (94%) and low infection rates, even in high-risk patient populations or complex trauma cases.
- SEFM may reduce complications such as dehiscence and mitigate the need for advanced reconstruction, making it valuable in managing challenging soft-tissue injuries.

INTRODUCTION

Soft-tissue management is a critical component of orthopedic reconstruction following traumatic injury.[1] Contamination, tissue loss, disrupted vascular supply, and presence of internal fixation are all common conditions that may limit soft-tissue reconstruction options and negatively impact successful surgical wound healing.[2] Tissue flap procedures, such as local rotational flaps and free flaps, are often considered as a means of providing wound coverage and vascularity to the site of injury.[3] These procedures, however, are not always feasible when considering the type of injury, available surgeons, and overall patient health status.[1,3,4] Local advancement or rotational flaps may be limited by insufficient availability of viable wound-adjacent tissue.[1–4] Free tissue transfer procedures require specialized surgeons to perform the procedure in addition to extensive operating time.[1] The availability of trained microsurgeons is a limiting factor for performing these procedures, in addition to patients who may have compromised vascularity due to trauma or chronic conditions and otherwise physiologically poor candidates for free tissue transfer.

Regenerative tissue matrices have been used clinically in orthopedic reconstruction to both stimulate healing responses and provide acute subcutaneous mechanical support postoperatively. Many existing materials are limited by their versatility in this setting. Biologic-based materials may be less than ideal for application in traumatic wounds that are contaminated at baseline due to elevated infection risk in a potentially colonized wound bed.[5] Furthermore, many of these materials are solely designed for topical use to stimulate dermal regeneration in open wound beds and require subsequent definitive closure through

[a] Department of Trauma, Campbell Clinic Orthopedics, Memphis, TN, USA; [b] Acera Surgical, Inc, St Louis, MO, USA
* Corresponding author. UT Department of Orthopaedic Surgery, Campbell Clinic, 1211 Union Avenue, Suite 500, Memphis, TN 38104.
E-mail address: ccosgrove@campbellclinic.com

Orthop Clin N Am 57 (2026) 329–338
https://doi.org/10.1016/j.ocl.2026.05.006
0030-5898/26/

Abbreviations	
BKA	below-knee amputation
CFUs	colony forming units
CKD	chronic kidney disease
COPD	chronic obstructive pulmonary disease
DM	diabetes mellitus
ECM	extracellular matrix
ESRD	end-stage renal disease
FDA	Food and Drug Administration
ISO	International Organization for Standardization
NPWT	negative pressure wound therapy
ORIF	open reduction and internal fixation
PAD	peripheral artery disease
PVD	peripheral vascular disease
SEFMs	synthetic electrospun fiber materials
STSG	split-thickness skin graft
TMAs	transmetatarsal amputations
USP	United States Pharmacopeia

autografting as opposed to offering regenerative support for damaged, but primarily closed, tissue.

Electrospun synthetic polymers have a growing area of interest for regenerative medicine due to their customizability, biocompatibility, and mechanical strength.[6] Synthetic polymers can be tailored to resemble that of native extracellular matrix (ECM) and thus facilitate wound healing responses on a cellular level through topographic rather than biochemical responses.[6,7] Polyglactin, for example, is a highly porous polymer that encourages cellular diffusion, neovascularization, and cellular attachment in addition to providing a high degree of mechanical strength.[8] One approach to customizing these polymers for clinical applications is through electrospinning. Solvent-based electrospinning utilizes a high voltage electric field, which creates a fiber jet between a needle and a charged polymer solution source, then depositing the newly formed fibers on a collector.[6,9] Electrospinners are highly customizable and provide a high degree of accuracy in adjusting the size and distribution of the fibers. As such, electrospun polymeric matrices can be engineered to resemble native ECM in both size and structure and ensure consistent quality of the materials produced.[6]

The unique advantages of synthetic, eletrospun polymers offer in terms of both tissue regeneration and reinforcement have been successfully translated to clinical use.[6–9] A synthetic electrospun fiber materials (SEFM; Restrata, Acera Surgical, Inc, St. Louis, Mo) received Food and Drug Administration (FDA) 510(k) clearance for 2 separate clinical indications: (1) as a wound healing device to encourage cellular infiltration and vascularization in a variety of both chronic and acute wounds, including partial/full-thickness wounds, ulcers, surgical wounds, and traumatic wounds and (2) as a soft-tissue reinforcement device for implantation to areas of soft-tissue weakness in patients requiring soft-tissue repair or reinforcement in reconstructive surgery.

The versatility of SEFM to be utilized either topically or subcutaneously could provide orthopedic trauma surgeons with an additional tool for utilization in complex soft-tissue injuries.[4] Extensive soft-tissue damage can present challenges in reconstruction such as insufficient tissue for primary surgical closure, increased infection risk, lack of coverage over exposed structures or orthopedic instrumentation, and tenuous surgical closures due to tension or a degloved dermal-epidermal structure. SEFM offers topical wound management support for remaining postsurgical wounds in which there was insufficient viable tissue surrounding the defect to provide adequate coverage.[4] In addition to supporting wound healing responses, SEFM also provides immediate wound coverage. Throughout the resorption process, SEFM encourages both regeneration of dermal tissues and re-epithelialization of quality, organized tissue, thus allowing for the surgeon and patient to determine an appropriate plan for closure, whether this be through subsequent skin grafting or permitting complete re-epithelialization through secondary intention wound healing.[4]

These features and indications of SEFM may offer a versatile solution to the various challenges associated with soft-tissue injury following orthopedic reconstructive surgery. This review aims to highlight existing preclinical and clinical data regarding SEFM use in orthopedic reconstruction and summarize the clinical efficacy of the device across a variety surgical procedures and injuries to date, as well as provide recommendations for further research of SEFM in this clinical specialty.

CURRENT EVIDENCE

The SEFM (Restrata , Acera Surgical, Inc, St. Louis, Mo) discussed herein is composed of 2 synthetic polymers (polyglactin 910 and polydioxanone), which are electrospun to create a

3 dimensional, nonwoven matrix.[6,9] These polymers create a fully synthetic matrix with various fiber diameters designed to elicit wound healing responses on a cellular level as well as provide a degree of tensile and mechanical strength similar to that of human skin.[6,9] SEFM is available in full sheet and premeshed configurations for application as both a topical wound healing device and subcutaneous soft-tissue reinforcement device. An additional configuration of SEFM is available in a particulate form (Restrata MiniMatrix, Acera Surgical, Inc, St. Louis, Mo) as a topical wound healing device and is particularly beneficial for easy application to areas of wound tunneling or undermining. All form factors of SEFM fully resorb roughly 28 days after application.

Preclinical Studies

Various preclinical investigations, both in vitro and in vivo, have been conducted on SEFM to date. These investigations have been conducted to evaluate SEFM's biocompatibility and efficacy as both a wound healing matrix and a soft-tissue reinforcement device.[7,10–12]

Wound healing and tissue quality

In an in vivo model evaluating overall healing outcomes in Yucatan miniature swine, SEFM was compared to a bilayered xenograft material in the treatment of full-thickness wounds.[7] Wound tissues harvested on day 15 and day 30 timepoints underwent semiqualitative histopathology analysis of hematoxylin and eosin stained slides per International Organization for Standardization (ISO) 10993-6 standards.[7] SEFM-treated tissues demonstrated less inflammation and more complete wound healing at both day 15 and day 30.[7] At day 15, SEFM-treated wounds demonstrated complete dermal regeneration of the wound area as compared to the bilayer xenograft matrix, in which regenerated tissue covered roughly 20% to 50% of the total wound area.[7]

Mechanical strength

Both in vivo and in vitro testing of SEFM was conducted to assess mechanical strength and biocompatibility as a means of obtaining FDA 510 (k) clearance for soft-tissue reinforcement in areas of soft-tissue weakness.[10] Testing included evaluation of tensile strength, burst strength, biocompatibility, and resorption rate against a substantially equivalent fish-skin product as a predicate.[10] In vitro testing of burst strength after 72 hours of preconditioning demonstrated that the SEFM was 23 times stronger than the predicate device.[11] In vivo outcomes in a porcine model provided further validity to benchtop results, demonstrating that SEFM-reinforced tissues were 49% stronger at day 3% and 21% stronger at day 10 when compared to fish skin-reinforced tissues.[11] Overall, in vivo tensile strength of SEFM remained similar to human skin for 7 to 10 days postimplantation.[10,11]

Antimicrobial effectiveness

Benchtop testing per United States Pharmacopeia (USP) <51> standards for Antimicrobial Effectiveness was performed on both particulate and sheet configurations of SEFM.[12] Testing was performed against the most common microbes found in nonhealing surgical wounds, which included *Escherichia coli*, *Pseudomonas aeruginosa*, *Staphylococcus aureus*, *Aspergillus brasiliensis*, *Candida albicans*, *Proteus mirabilis*, and *Enterococcus faecalis*.[12] Following initial exposure to these microbes, testing at days 7, 14, and 28 was performed to measure the presence of colony forming units (CFU).[12] The sheet configuration demonstrated greater than 3-log_{10} reduction to no detectable colonies of *E coli*, *S aureus*, *P aeruginosa*, *P mirabilis*, *E faecalis*, and *C albicans* at day 14 and 28, with no increase of *A brasiliensis* from the time of initial inoculation.[12] The particulate configuration demonstrated a greater than 3-log_{10} reduction to no detectable colonies of all microorganisms at day 7.[12] These results indicated that, in vitro, SEFM is effective and inhibiting bacterial and fungal growth per USP <51> testing.

Clinical Outcomes

SEFM has been studied clinically across a variety of chronic and acute wound etiologies to date in the form of case reports, case series, retrospective studies, prospective studies, and randomized controlled trials.[13–20]

Clinical results in chronic and acute wounds

Chronic wounds including diabetic foot ulcers venous leg ulcers have demonstrated high rates of wound closure with minimal complications.[13–15] Acute wounds, including hidradenitis suppurativa excisions, soft-tissue trauma, soft-tissue infections, cancer excisions, and head and neck reconstructions have also demonstrated clinical success following SEFM application with no published instances of infection to date.[16–20] Published studies in acute wound care have demonstrated versatility of SEFM application as it encourages both dermal and epidermal regeneration, allowing for either staged closure with skin-grafting or complete re-epithelialization through secondary intention healing.

Clinical Outcomes in Orthotrauma

SEFM application in orthopedic trauma cases has been studied through a variety of case reports and retrospective reviews evaluating the various types of injury etiologies that have been treated, as well as the mode of application (topical or subdermal).[21–29]

Clinical histology

Histology of tissues regenerated with SEFM has been studied in a clinical setting. A patient with numerous traumatic injuries resulting from a motor vehicle accident developed a nonhealing wound on the heel with exposed calcaneus despite numerous attempts at coverage.[21] SEFM was utilized as a salvage therapy after 2 years of multiple attempted treatments and recurrent infections. Multiple SEFM applications over 7 months successfully supported tissue regeneration over the exposed calcaneus; however, the patient eventually elected to undergo a below-knee amputation (BKA) due to pain and functional disability from posttraumatic ankle arthritis.[21] The patient consented to having the heel region and bone with regenerated tissue sent for histologic evaluation. Evaluation was conducted utilizing ISO 10993-6 standards, which demonstrated mild acute inflammation, moderate new vascularization, and moderate organized collagen deposition.[21] At the bone/tissue interface, no evidence of necrosis or bacterial colonization was observed.[21]

Synthetic electrospun fiber material in traumatic wound management

SEFM has been applied topically to a variety of injury etiologies in both general trauma and orthopedic trauma to date, including soft-tissue degloving, crush injuries, open fractures, traumatic amputation, and fasciotomies.[22–25] In these instances, primary closure of the injury was not feasible considering the size of the defect. In consideration of both injury etiology and patient health status, SEFM was utilized to either (1) prepare the wound bed for subsequent STSG application by stimulating regeneration of viable tissue in wounds with exposed structures or uneven contour or (2) encourage complete re-epithelialization through secondary intention healing (**Fig. 1**). To date, a total of 14 patients across 4 publications have been treated with SEFM topically to manage musculoskeletal soft-tissue trauma injuries.[22–25] **Table 1** provides an overview of relevant publications.

Many authors have employed negative pressure wound therapy (NPWT) as a bolster in conjunction with SEFM for the first 10 to 14 days postoperatively, followed by application of nonadherent dressings following NPWT takedown. This approach ensures that the SEFM remains in full contact with the wound bed, which is critical to maximizing the effectiveness of SEFM.[22–25]

Most of these studies report using only a single application of SEFM to achieve desired healing outcomes. Secondary intention healing was utilized in 3 patients. Tacconi and colleagues[24] utilized SEFM to achieve secondary intention healing of a traumatic soft-tissue degloving injury in an elderly patient with multiple comorbidities, including advanced liver cirrhosis, protein-calorie, malnutrition, and a history of osteomyelitis, which made her a poor candidate for autografting. Cosgrove utilized secondary intention healing to achieve closure in 1 patient with an open foot crush injury and another patient who underwent a decompressive fasciotomy for forearm compartment syndrome, both of whom were active smokers throughout treatment.[25] The average time to complete re-epithelialization for these patients was 11.9 weeks with no instances of infection or other wound complications.[22–25]

The majority of publications to date report on utilization of SEFM as a means supporting dermal regeneration for subsequent skin grafting.[22,23,25] This approach has been utilized in crush injuries, soft-tissue degloving injuries, traumatic amputation, and both upper and lower extremity open fractures. The median time from SEFM application to skin-grafting across these publications is reported to be around 4.1 weeks, with an average STSG take rate of 98%.[22,23,25] No instances of skin-graft loss or infection have been reported to date.[22–25]

Synthetic electrospun fiber material in acute subcutaneous soft-tissue reinforcement

SEFM has also been successfully utilized subcutaneously in various orthopedic procedures as a means of providing soft-tissue reinforcement to areas of soft-tissue weakness.[26–29] This approach has been utilized a means to reduce the risk of dehiscence following primary closure in high-risk patients or procedures.[26–29] Published literature regarding subdermal application of SEFM investigates use in transmetatarsal amputations (TMAs), Achilles rupture repairs, bimalleolar and trimalleolar ankle fractures, open fractures, soft-tissue degloving injuries, traumatic amputations, and revision procedures.[26–29] To date, 46 patients have been treated across a total of 4

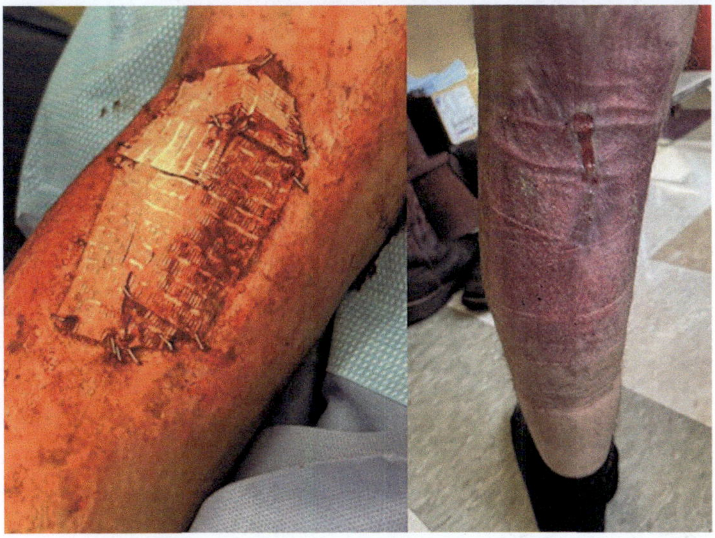

Fig. 1. An open traumatic wound in the popliteal fossa. Split-thickness skin graft application over a flexion crease is typically fraught with complications including contracture. SEFM allowed for the patient to continually move and perform physical therapy while healing through secondary intention, avoiding any knee flexion or extension contracture.

publications investigating the use of subdermal SEFM application as a means of reinforcing primary surgical closure (Table 2).

Subdermal SEFM application has been utilized as a means of mitigating dehiscence risk, augmenting skin flaps (Fig. 2), providing coverage over tendon or orthopedic implants, and offloading tenuous closures (Fig. 3).[28,29] Patient factors also are taken into account when considering the use of SEFM, as high-risk populations such as active smokers, elderly patients, or patients with uncontrolled diabetes mellitus or peripheral vascular disease are at increased risks of wound healing complications.[26–29]

In a TMA study conducted by Alexander and colleagues,[27] patients received SEFM application underlying the suture line during primary closure demonstrated improved healing outcomes compared to the control group. The SEFM-augmented group had higher rates of complete healing (80% vs 60%), decreased instances of dehiscence (5 vs 8), and decreased rates of limb loss (20% vs 40%).[27] Positive healing outcomes have also been observed in Barton and colleagues' study, in which 100% of augmented TMA's achieved complete closure with one instance of wound dehiscence.[26] In both Alexander's and Barton's studies, TMAs

Table 1
Current publications and key outcomes associated with topical synthetic electrospun fiber material application in musculoskeletal trauma injuries

Authors	Injury Etiology(s) (n)	Location of Injury(s) (n)	Wound Closure Approach (n)	Wound Closure Achieved (%)	Surgical Site Infection (n)
Martini et al,[22] 2022	Crush injury (1)	Dorsal foot (1)	STSG[a] (1)	100%	0
Fernandez et al,[23] 2024	Soft-tissue degloving (1)	Groin/thigh (1)	STSG (1)	100%	0
Tacconi, et al,[24] 2025	Soft-tissue degloving (1)	Forearm (1)	Secondary intention (1)	100%	0
Cosgrove[25] 2025	Open fracture (7) Crush injury (2) Traumatic amputation (1) Fasciotomy (1)	Lower extremity (4) Forearm (4) Foot (3)	STSG (8) Secondary intention (2)	91%	1 (NPWT[b] malfunction)

[a] STSG, split-thickness skin graft.
[b] NPWT, negative pressure wound therapy.

Table 2
Current publications and key outcomes associated with subdermal synthetic electrospun fiber material application for soft-tissue reinforcement in orthopedic surgery

Authors	Injury/Surgical Etiology(s) (n)	Location of Injury(s) (n)	Clinical Indication for SEFM Application (n)	Wound Closure Achieved (%)	Surgical Site Infection (n)
Alexander et al,[27] 2022	Transmetatarsal amputation (10)	Forefoot (10)	High-risk patient population with diagnoses including DM[a], PVD[b], and ESRD[c]	80%	0
Barton and Abicht [26] 2021	Transmetatarsal amputation (7)	Forefoot (7)	High-risk patient population with diagnoses included DM, PAD[d], COPD[e], and CKD[f]	100%	0
Rushing [28] 2023	Achilles rupture (1) Trimalleolar ankle fracture (1) Bimalleolar ankle fracture (3) Revision procedure (1) Pressure injury (2) Arthrodesis (1) Medial malleolus fracture (1)	Ankle (8) Foot (2)	Dehiscence risk (4) Implant coverage (1) Patient history of poor healing (2) Patient comorbidities (2) Augment skin flap (1)	100%	1
Cosgrove [29] 2026	Open fracture (11) Revision procedure (4) Soft-tissue degloving (2) Traumatic amputation (1) Achilles rupture repair (1)	Lower extremity (15) Upper extremity (4)	Tenuous closure (10) Augment skin flap (4) Tendon coverage (4) Implant coverage (4)	100%	1

[a] DM, diabetes mellitus.
[b] PVD, peripheral vascular disease.
[c] ESRD, end-stage renal disease.
[d] PAD, peripheral artery disease.
[e] COPD, chronic obstructive pulmonary disease.
[f] CKD, chronic kidney disease.

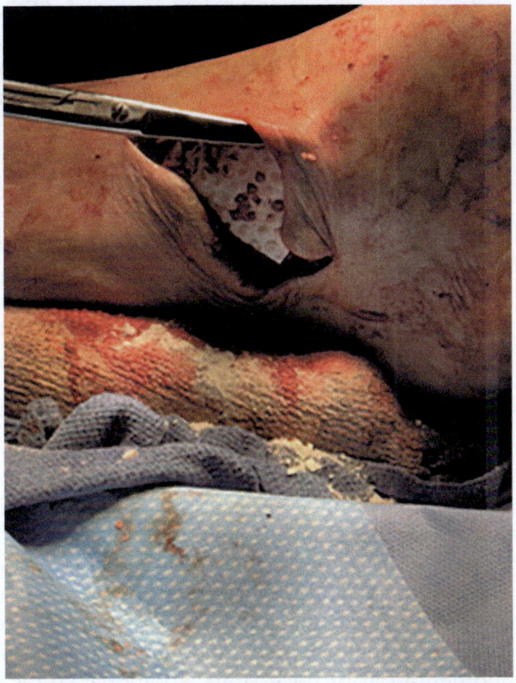

Fig. 2. A degloved medial ankle wound following an open-fracture dislocation. A full sheet of SEFM is applied underlying the devitalized epidermis to support primary closure.

were performed due to nonhealing ulcers as a result of diabetes mellitus or peripheral vascular disease.[26,27] Given these patients' comorbidities and history of nonhealing, SEFM was incorporated into primary closure as a way of encouraging successful closure and reducing healing complications in this high-risk population.

Cosgrove[29] and Rushing[28] utilized SEFM as means to support primary closure of fractures (both open and closed), Achilles rupture repairs, soft-tissue degloving injuries, and revision procedures. SEFM was utilized as a means to provide mechanical offloading during tenuous primary closure, which successfully mitigated the need for more advanced reconstructive procedures.[29] SEFM was also utilized as a barrier between the suture line and nearby hardware or tendon as a means of mitigating the risk of exposed structures if dehiscence were to occur.[28,29] All patients in both studies achieved complete epidermal closure of their surgical sites.[28,29] There were 2 instances of superficial surgical infection (SSIs) which were operatively managed, and both patients went on to fully heal without further complications.[28,29] In Cosgrove's study, 5 patients experienced minor superficial wound breakdown; however, initial study findings suggest that subdermal SEFM application likely played a role in minimizing the severity of these complications, which were successfully managed with local wound care and did not necessitate reoperation.[29]

DISCUSSION

Infection is among the largest threats to successful healing in orthopedic surgery. The rate of deep SSI following open reduction and internal fixation (ORIF) of bimalleolar ankle fractures has been reported to be as high as 19% in one study, with a majority of these patients necessitating hardware removal.[30] *S aureus* represents the most common cause of post-ORIF infections of the ankle, with 1 study identifying a 17% BKA rate following infection.[31] Open fractures generally present with a greater infection rate due to compromised skin barriers and extensive soft-tissue trauma.[32] The rate of SSIs for closed fractures is around 2% to 5% and increases by 50%

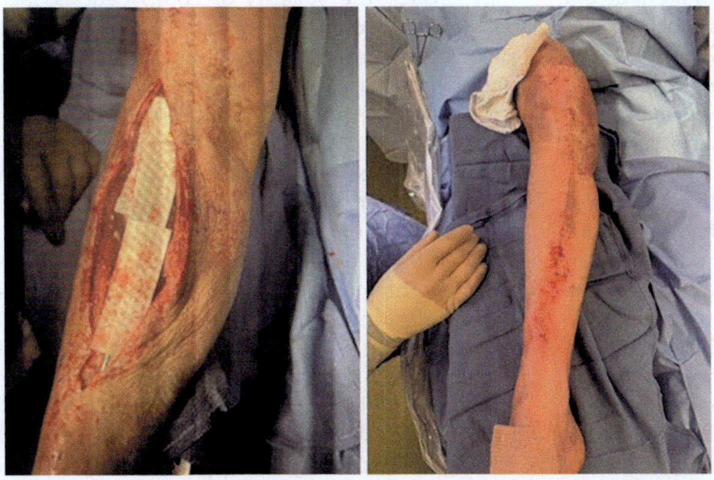

Fig. 3. An anterior tibia surgical wound reinforced with SEFM underlying primary closure.

for patients who experience open fractures.[32] Revision procedures performed to address poor outcomes following primary intervention for traumatic injuries also present a high risk of infection, particularly in the lower extremity.[33] These procedures have a reported SSI rate of around 17% and a deep SSI rate of around 10% as reported in one 2 year retrospective review.[33] Furthermore, patients who developed deep SSIs required an average of 2.6 surgical procedures, with 33% eventually necessitating amputation.[33]

In addition to increased patient morbidity and mortality, postoperative complications also result in increased cost of care.[34] A cost of care analysis conducted by Healy and colleagues[34] reported that mean hospital costs were 119% higher in patients who experienced postoperative complications as compared to patients without complications. A subanalysis of SSI-related complications showed that superficial SSIs resulted in a 37% increase in resource costs used by the hospital, and a 42% increase for deep SSIs.[34] A review of costs associated with ankle fractures alone reported that 12 month incremental commercial payments in patients who experienced infection or reoperation were US$27,510 and US$13,577, respectively.[35]

Postoperative healing complications are more likely to occur in older patients with multiple comorbidities.[34] Risk factors for healing complications such as SSIs most often include tobacco dependency, hypertension, obesity, and diabetes mellitus.[34,36–38] In the present review, patients who received SEFM application for the management of a variety of orthopedic trauma injuries, including revisions and both open and closed fractures, had an estimated 5% infection rate. This is notable when considering 53% of the combined population across both of Cosgrove's publications were active smokers at the time of surgery, and 17% had a diagnosis of diabetes mellitus.[25,29] Reduction of SSIs is critical to improving patient outcomes as well as reducing total cost of care. One study reviewing costs associated with the treatment of infected fractures revealed additional costs of US$19,125 for superficial SSIs and US$40,289 for deep SSIs.[32] An initial review of published literature on SEFM use shows promising outcomes in reduction of SSIs, especially among patients with risk factors for poor healing outcomes.[22–29] SEFM's passing results per USP <51> testing of Antimicrobial Efficacy may provide some context for these observed outcomes, particularly against *S aureus*, which is the leading cause of infection post-ORIF ankle fractures.[12,31]

A review of literature to date regarding SEFM application in traumatic injuries demonstrates a degree of versatility and low complication profile that is highly valuable in soft-tissue reconstruction following orthopedic trauma.[22–29] Multiple product configurations and indications for use allow for a greater degree in tailoring soft-tissue reconstruction to the individual patient in consideration of overall patient health, degree of injury, and availability of surrounding viable tissues. Clinical outcomes to date demonstrate a low infection rate and an overall 94% complete closure rate across amputation sites, revision procedures, degloving injuries, Achilles rupture repairs, and both open and closed fractures.[32]

A review of current publications demonstrates successful use of SEFM underlying primary closure during orthopedic repairs.[28,29] Use of SEFM as a means of offloading tension at the surgical site permitted for primary closure of open fracture injuries that may have otherwise been at significant risk of dehiscence without augmentation or necessitate additional surgical interventions to achieve complete closure.[29] Preclinical studies of SEFM have demonstrated its ability to maintain its tensile strength for up to 10 days postoperatively, which is critical when considering the majority of wound dehiscence incidents occur 5 to 10 days postoperatively.[11] As demonstrated in Alexander and colleagues' study, augmented TMAs experienced less occurrences of wound dehiscence, less instances of limb loss, and a higher rate of complete closure.[27] While minor occurrences of dehiscence occurred in Cosgrove's patient population, they were all superficial and presented without evidence of infection, thus were able to be managed with local wound care at bedside.[29] Subdermal applications of SEFM may reduce the severity of complications such as surgical wound dehiscence by providing a protective barrier between the suture line and underlying hardware as well as by augmenting the strength of the sutured tissues.[10] Reduction in severity of complications both improves patient outcomes and reduces total cost of care by avoiding additional cost and risk associated with reoperation.

While initial outcomes observed in SEFM management of musculoskeletal injuries are promising, utilization of SEFM in this area of clinical practice is somewhat novel. Given the novelty of this treatment approach, publications on the clinical use of SEFM to date are limited by retrospective study designs and a wide variety of wound etiologies and surgical approaches. This can create challenges of elucidating the exact effects of SEFM use and soft-tissue healing outcomes. Future studies should explore SEFM outcomes associated with specific injuries or surgical procedures in a large patient cohort with a control population for comparison of results.

SUMMARY

SEFM is a fully synthetic, electrospun, polymer wound matrix with indications as both a wound healing device and as a subdermal soft-tissue reinforcement device. The synthetic composition of the matrix as well as its versatility in clinical applications may provide a unique tool in improving outcomes following orthopedic trauma. Both preclinical and clinical outcomes observed in a review of published literature to date demonstrate success in promoting soft-tissue healing, with a high rate of complete closure and low rates of SSIs or other major complications. Further research regarding the utility of SEFM in orthopedic trauma reconstruction should be conducted to identify ideal scenarios for clinical use.

CLINICS CARE POINTS

- Traumatic wounds with orthopedic injuries have a high complication profile, including infection, nonunion and soft-tissue breakdown requiring local or free tissue flaps, or amputation.
- SEFM resembles native ECM and provides a structure on which cellular infiltration and proliferation may quickly mature a wound bed.
- SEFM has been used successfully in both open wounds as well as subcutaneously to promote soft-tissue reinforcement of a primary, but tenuous, skin closure.
- SEFM has met Antimicrobial Effectiveness criteria per in vitro USP-51 testing demonstrating a greater than 3-log reduction in 7 common wound microbes over 28 day period.
- Future rigorous trials are needed to establish clinical benefit; reduction of infection rates, soft-tissue coverage requirements, in the orthopedic trauma population.

DISCLOSURE

C. Cosgrove is a paid consultant for Acera Surgical, Inc, and received compensation for time spent on article preparation. E. Sallade is an employee of and has stock options with Acera Surgical, Inc.

REFERENCES

1. Holler JT, Albright P, Challa S, et al. Barriers to performing soft tissue reconstruction among orthopedic surgeons in low- and middle-income countries: results of a surgical skills training course. Plastic Reconstr Surg Glob Open 2019;7(10):e2420.
2. Moola FO, Alberto A, Berry GK, et al. Attempting primary closure for all open fractures: the effectiveness of an institutional protocol. Can J Surg 2014; 57:E82–8.
3. Koster ITS, Borgdorff MP, Jamaludin FS, et al. Strategies following free flap failure in lower extremity trauma: a systematic review. JPRAS Open 2023; 36:94–104.
4. Cosgrove C. Soft tissue reconstruction with synthetic electrospun fiber matrix following musculoskeletal injury: a retrospective case series. Eplasty 2025;25:e37.
5. Nair A, Dahiya A, Yadav P, et al. Materials for the management of traumatic wounds: a descriptive review. Eur Polym J 2025;222:112475.
6. MacEwan M, Jeng L, Kovacs T, et al. Clinical application of bioresorbable, synthetic, electrospun matrix in wound healing. Bioengineering (Basel) 2022; 10(1):9.
7. MacEwan MR, MacEwan S, Wright AP, et al. Comparison of a fully synthetic electrospun matrix to a bilayered xenograft in healing full thickness cutaneous wounds in a porcine model. Cureus 2017;9(8):e1614.
8. Lesko L, Jungova P, Culenova M, et al. Polymer-based scaffolds as an implantable material in regenerative dentistry: a review. J Funct Biomater 2025;16(3):80.
9. MacEwan MR, MacEwan S, Kovacs TR, et al. What makes the optimal wound healing material? A review of current science and introduction of a synthetic nanofabricated wound care scaffold. Cureus 2017;9(10):e1736.
10. U.S. Food and Drug Administration, 510(k) Premarket Notification. Restrata soft tissue reinforcement (STR) K251224 premarket notification. 2025. Available at: https://www.accessdata.fda.gov/cdrh_docs/pdf25/K251224.pdf. Accessed November 10, 2025.
11. Acera Surgical, Inc. Restrata electrospun fiber matrix platform technology (Brochure). 2025.
12. Sallade E, Grimes D, Jeng L, et al. Antimicrobial effectiveness testing of resorbable electrospun fiber matrix per United States Pharmacoepia (USP) <51>. Cureus 2023;15(12):e50055.
13. Regulski MJ, MacEwan MR. Implantable nanomedical scaffold facilitates healing of chronic lower extremity wounds. Wounds 2018;30(8):E77–80.
14. Abicht BP, Deitrick GA, MacEwan MR, et al. Evaluation of wound healing of diabetic foot ulcers in a prospective clinical trial using a synthetic hybrid-scale fiber matrix. Foot Ankle Surg 2022;2(1):100135.

15. Husain K, Malik A, Kirchens J, et al. A prospective, blinded, randomized controlled clinical trial evaluating the effect of the synthetic electrospun fiber matrix in the treatment of chronic diabetic foot ulcers. Foot Ankle Surg 2024;4(1):100362.
16. Madueke M, Lau F. Synthetic electrospun fiber matrix in the management of acute wound following excision of hidradenitis suppurativa lesions: a prospective pilot study. Polymers 2025; 17(19):2563.
17. Fernandez L, Kim PJ, Williams N, et al. Synthetic hybrid-scale fiber matrix in the trauma and acute care surgical practice. Wounds 2021;33(9): 237–44.
18. McGowan J. Reconstruction of post-mohs surgical wounds using a novel nanofiber matrix. Wounds 2022;34(8):209–15.
19. Zaiac M, Kauffman M, Matin T, et al. Utility of synthetic hybrid-scale fiber matrix in dermatologic wounds. JAAD Case Rep 2023;40:109–11.
20. Horwich P, Sivarajah S, Neskey D, et al. Applications of synthetic hybrid-scale fiber matrix in head and neck reconstruction: a case series. Case Rep Oncol 2024;17(1):622–9.
21. Harder JG, Hernandez EJ, MacEwan M, et al. Histopathologic analysis of a recalcitrant calcaneal wound treated using a synthetic hybrid-scale fiber matrix. Plastic Reconstr Surg Glob Open 2024; 12(2):e5597.
22. Martini CJ, Burgess B, Ghodasra JH. Treatment of traumatic crush injury using a synthetic hybrid-scale fiber matrix in conjunction with split-thickness skin graft. Foot Ankle Surg 2022;2(1): 100112.
23. Fernandez LG, Matthews MR, Norwood S, et al. Synergistic clinical application of synthetic electrospun fiber wound matrix in the management of a complex traumatic wound: degloving left groin and thigh auger injury. Wounds 2024;36(4): 124–8.
24. Tacconi KA, Deering AJ, Malekpour M, et al. Novel use of synthetic elctrospun wound matrix in an extensive forearm degloving injury: case report and review of the literature. Plastic Reconstr Surg Glob Open 2025;13(9):e7094.
25. Cosgrove C. Soft tissue reconstruction with synthetic electrospun fiber matrix following musculoskeletal injury: a retrospective case series. Eplasty 2025;25:e37.
26. Barton EC, Abicht BP. Lower extremity wounds treated with a synthetic hybrid-scale fiber matrix. Foot Ankle Surg 2021;1(3):100076.
27. Alexander J, Desai V, Denden S, et al. Assessment of a novel augmented closure technique for surgical wounds associated with transmetatarsal amputation: a preliminary study. J Am Podiatry Assoc 2022;112(5):20–256.
28. Rushing CJ. Lower extremity orthopedic augmentation utilizing a synthetic hybrid-scale fiber matrix. Cureus 2023;15(9):e45046.
29. Cosgrove C. Pilot study: soft-tissue healing after augmented closure of traumatic injuries with synthetic electrospun fiber matrix. Plastic Reconstr Surg Glob Open 2026;14(3):e7557.
30. Thangarajah T, Prasad PSV, Narayan B. Surgical site infections following open reduction and internal fixation of ankle fractures. Open Orthop J 2009;3: 56–60.
31. Zalavras CG, Christensen T, Rigopoulos N, et al. Infection following operative treatment of ankle fractures. Clin Orthop Relat Res 2009;467(7):1715–20.
32. O'Connor O, Thahir A, Krkovic M. How much does an infected fracture cost? Arch Bone Jt Surg 2022; 10(2):135–40.
33. Heinz NR, Clement ND, Young RN, et al. Rate and factors associated with surgical site infection following aseptic revision fixation of orthopaedic trauma injuries. Eur J Orthop Surg Traumatol 2023;33(8):3511–7.
34. Healy MA, Mullard AJ, Campbell DA Jr, et al. Hospital and payer costs associated with surgical complications. JAMA Surg 2016;151(9):823–30.
35. Vanderkarr MF, Ruppenkamp JW, Vanderkarr M, et al. Incidence, costs and post-operative complication following ankle fracture- A US claims database analysis. BMC Musculoskelet Disord 2022;23:1129.
36. Sagherian BH, Hoballah JJ, Tamim H. Comparing the 30-day complications between smokers and non-smokers undergoing surgical fixation of ankle fractures. Foot Ankle Orthop 2022;7(3):24730114221115677.
37. Hanlon M, Horner O, Kenny F, et al. Obesity and trauma. In: O'Byrne JM, Rowan F, Molloy A, editors. Musculoskeletal disease and obesity. Cham: Springer; 2024.
38. Stolarczyk A, Sarzynska S, Gondek A, et al. Influence of diabetes on tissue healing in orthopaedic injuries. Clin Exp Pharmacol Physiol 2018;45(7): 619–27.

Transverse Tibial Transport for Limb Salvage in Ischemic Lower Extremity Disease

Technique, Mechanisms, and Clinical Outcomes—A Systematic Review

Samuel Raszka, MD, Max Michalski, MD, MS, Charles Moon, MD*

KEYWORDS

- Transverse tibial transport • Diabetic foot ulcer • Chronic limb-threatening ischemia
- Limb salvage • Distraction osteogenesis

KEY POINTS

- Transverse tibial transport (TTT) stimulates angiogenesis and microcirculatory regeneration, addressing the microvascular component of ischemic lower extremity disease that macrovascular repair alone cannot correct.
- Meta-analysis from Hu et al reports wound healing and limb salvage rates of 0.96 and 0.98 with healing OR of 10.43 vs non TTT controls.
- TTT with endovascular therapy improves amputation free survival at 12 and 24 months vs endovascular therapy aloneTTT is reproducible without the need for specialized.
- TTT is reproducible without the need for specialized preopeative imaging. Purpose-built systems and guides are now commercially available in the United Stataes.
- Further high-quality prospective randomized trials and health economic analyses are required to standardize protocols and define TTT's optimal role within multidisciplinary limb salvage care pathways.

INTRODUCTION

Chronic limb-threatening ischemia (CLTI) and diabetic foot ulcers (DFUs) represent an escalating global health crisis. Diabetes mellitus affects an estimated 536.6 million people worldwide, a figure projected to reach 783.2 million by 2045. Of those with diabetes, 19% to 34% will develop a foot ulcer during their lifetime, and more than 15% of DFUs will necessitate lower extremity amputation, making this the most common cause of nontraumatic limb loss globally.[1,2] Beyond diabetes, thromboangiitis obliterans, peripheral arterial disease, vasculitis, and venous insufficiency further contribute to the spectrum of ischemic lower extremity ulceration.[3]

Despite significant advances in endovascular therapy (EVT) and open surgical revascularization, many patients fail to achieve durable wound healing due to persistent microvascular disease. Even after successful restoration of large-vessel inflow, foot microperfusion frequently remains impaired and ulcers may fail to heal or recur at high rates. Studies suggest that 30% to 50% of patients with severe DFUs are unsuitable candidates for revascularization due to comorbidities or anatomy, yet standard wound care alone achieves healing rates as low as 40% to 60%.[4,5]

Department of Orthopaedic Surgery, Cedars-Sinai Medical Center, Los Angeles, CA, USA
* Corresponding author. Department of Orthopaedic Surgery, Cedars Sinai Orthopaedic Center, 444 S San Vicente Boulevard, Suite 603, Los Angeles, CA 90048.
E-mail address: Charles.Moon@cshs.org

Orthop Clin N Am 57 (2026) 339–348
https://doi.org/10.1016/j.ocl.2026.05.007

Abbreviations	
3D	3 dimensional
95%CI	95% confidence interval
AFS	amputation-free survival
CLTI	chronic limb-threatening ischemia
CT	computed tomography
DFUs	diabetic foot ulcers
EVT	endovascular therapy
FDA	Food and Drug Administration
TAO	thromboangiitis obliterans
$TcPO_2$	transcutaneous oxygen pressure
TTT	transverse tibial transport
VEGF	vascular endothelial growth factor

Transverse tibial transport (TTT)—also termed tibial cortex transverse transport or tibial cortex transverse distraction—has emerged as a novel adjunctive surgical strategy that addresses microvascular dysfunction through mechanobiologic stimulation. Rather than operating on the ischemic wound itself, TTT creates a cortical bone window in the proximal tibia and distracts it transversely using an external fixator, triggering a systemic cascade of angiogenic, immunomodulatory, and regenerative responses that translate into improved distal limb perfusion and wound healing without directly manipulating macrovascular anatomy.[6,7]

The conceptual foundation of TTT traces to Ilizarov's 1989 investigations demonstrating that gradual tissue distraction promotes regeneration of bone, vasculature, and soft tissue through the "law of tension-stress."[4] The first clinical application specifically for ischemic ulceration was reported in 2001 for thromboangiitis obliterans.[18] Over subsequent decades, the technique has undergone substantial refinement—from bulky ring fixators to dedicated unilateral systems—and achieved expert consensus formalization in 2020.[19] Regulatory clearance has since been obtained in the European Union and the United States,[20] heralding broader international adoption.

This systematic review synthesizes evidence from 35 source publications, ranging from multicenter prospective cohort studies to case series, to provide a comprehensive reference on TTT for clinicians and researchers engaged in lower extremity limb salvage (Table 1).

BIOLOGIC RATIONALE AND MECHANISM

The therapeutic effects of TTT originate from Ilizarov's foundational law of tension-stress, which demonstrated that controlled mechanical distraction of living tissues promotes regeneration of bone, vasculature, and soft tissue.[4] Canine models of transverse tibial distraction confirmed that vessel volume in the distraction area increased more than 3 fold, and that blood flow increased up to 10 fold during active distraction before stabilizing at several times the baseline during consolidation. These observations underpinned the hypothesis—later validated clinically—that transverse tibial distraction would produce robust neovascularization extending to the distal ischemic limb.

Experimental and clinical investigations have identified multiple converging molecular pathways through which TTT exerts its angiogenic and regenerative effects. Growth factor signaling—particularly through vascular endothelial growth factor (VEGF) and hypoxia-inducible factor pathways—drives endothelial proliferation and new vessel formation. Serum VEGF levels increase approximately 2 fold following TTT in clinical series, and computed tomography (CT) angiography has confirmed marked neovascularization with increased small artery density and substantially elevated foot blood flow after surgery.[1,10] Endothelial progenitor cells are mobilized from the bone marrow into peripheral circulation and home to wound sites via growth factor gradients, contributing to neovascularization and re-epithelialization.[21,22]

Beyond angiogenesis, TTT exerts important immunomodulatory effects. Experimental models demonstrate a shift in wound macrophages from a proinflammatory toward a reparative phenotype, reducing cytokine-mediated tissue damage and improving the extracellular matrix environment for healing.[23] Multiomics proteomics studies in patients have shown that the upward distraction phase activates a broad systemic immune response, while wound closure occurs during the return phase—with 64.7% of patients requiring no antibiotics throughout the treatment course, suggesting meaningful anti-infective benefit.[24] Additional mechanisms include the release of small extracellular vesicles enriched with microRNAs and antioxidant proteins during bone transport, which accumulate at wound sites to mobilize fibroblasts, promote angiogenesis, and reduce oxidative stress.[25] The Ras/Raf/MEK/ERK kinase cascade and the osteopontin-nitric oxide axis have also been identified as mechanistic contributors linking tibial microinjury to vascular cell migration and wound repair.[15,26–29]

This mechanistic pluripotency—spanning angiogenic growth factor signaling, progenitor

Table 1
Key clinical studies and reviews of transverse tibial transport

Study	n	Indication	Key Outcomes	Complications
Chen et al,[5] 2020 (CORR) — landmark single-center series	249	Recalcitrant DFU (Texas 2C–3D)	96% healing; 97.1% limb salvage vs 77.4% control ($P<.001$); neovascularization on CTA	Low; no tibial fractures
Chen et al,[1] 2022 — multicenter prospective cohort (7 centers)	1175	Recalcitrant DFU (Texas 2C–3D)	94.9% healed; mean healing 12.4 wk; 4.9% major amputation; foot blood flow 8.1→28.3 mL/100 g/min; QoL improved	0.7% tibial fracture; 2.1% pin-site infection
Luxon et al,[2] 2025 — systematic review (13 studies)	924	Ischemic lower limb ulcers (predominantly DFU)	94% healed (TTT) vs 68% (control); ABI 0.54→0.88; VEGF 71→155 pg/mL; VAS 5→0–1	Pin-site infection (rare); tibial fracture n = 2
Hu et al,[8] 2023 — systematic review & meta-analysis (7 studies)	818	DFU	Pooled healing rate 0.96 (95%CI 0.93–0.98); limb salvage 0.98; ABI MD +0.23; VAS MD 3.70; recurrence RR 0.18 vs non-TTT ($P = .001$)	Fracture risk 0.02; pin-site infection 0.08
Ding et al,[3] 2024 — TTT + EVT vs EVT alone (CLTI)	131	CLTI (Rutherford 5+)	AFS at 12 mo: 81.9% (TTT + EVT) vs 48.9% (EVT); AFS at 24 mo: 74.2%; all surviving TTT + EVT patients achieved wound healing	Low; comparable to EVT alone
Qin et al,[9] 2023 — bilateral DFU PSM study	68	Bilateral DFU (Texas 2B–3D)	Healing 91.2% (UDFU) vs 76.5% (BDFU) at 1 y ($P = .10$); bilateral neovascularization confirmed by CTA from unilateral TTT	3 amputations; 2 recurrences
Liu et al,[10] 2024 (Frontiers Endocrinol) — modified TTT, 98 pts	98	DFU Wagner ≥II (dual-window modified)	95.83% healing; mean healing 53 d; ABI, WIFi, VAS all significantly improved at 3 mo; no recurrences	8.16% complication rate; no tibial fracture
Nie et al,[11] 2021 — non-diabetic leg ulcers	85	Recalcitrant nondiabetic leg ulcers (arterial, venous, and mixed)	78.6% healed (TTT) vs 58.1% (control) at 1 y (OR 2.64, $P = .04$); healing time 4.5 vs 6.1 mo ($P = .02$)	No skin necrosis; all osteotomy sites healed
Hong & Jin,[12] 2025 — thromboangiitis obliterans (119 pts)	119	Lower limb thromboangiitis obliterans (TAO)	TTT superior to conventional treatment in functional recovery, hemorheological parameters, QoL, and overall effectiveness	Not specifically quantified
Liu et al,[13] 2025 (Orthop Surg) — prognostic factors, 120 pts	120	DFU (various Wagner grades)	95% foot retention; 81.7% functional foot; combined 4 factor AUC = 0.998; independent risk factors: foot temp, $TcPO_2$, glucose, and CRP	Osteotomy necrosis 8.3%; DVT 5.8%; pin-tract 2.5%

(continued on next page)

Table 1
(continued)

Study	n	Indication	Key Outcomes	Complications
Jianda et al,[14] 2023 — large heel ulcers	21	Diabetic heel ulcers (mean 67 cm^2)	100% limb salvage; mean 128.6 d; 18 out of 21 walked independently	1 pin-site infection; 2 superficial ruptures
Wong et al,[7] 2025 — first international series (Singapore)	6	Refractory DFU (TTT as adjunct)	100% limb salvage and healing; median 4 mo; confirms reproducibility outside China	No pin-site infections
Zuo et al,[15] 2018 — chronic limb ischemia vs PTBA	90	TAO/arteriosclerotic occlusive disease	Larger artery diameters, higher blood flow, faster wound healing and pain resolution vs PTBA (all $P<.05$)	Not separately reported
Chang et al,[16] 2023 — integrated surgical wound treatment mode	13	DFU Wagner 3–4 (TTT + debridement + VSD + skin graft)	100% healed; no amputations; mean healing 25.8 d; CTA showed new arterial collateral network	1 pin channel infection; no serious complications
Wen et al,[17] 2023 (pilot study) — TTT vs conventional debridement	70	DFU Wagner ≥2 (35 TTT, 35 control)	TTT: significantly lower VAS, better ABI, lower MNSI neuropathy scores (all $P<.05$)	Not specifically reported

cell mobilization, immunomodulation, and paracrine vesicle release—distinguishes TTT from conventional surgical approaches focused solely on macrovascular correction and likely accounts for the robustness and durability of its clinical effects across diverse ischemic wound etiologies.

SURGICAL TECHNIQUE

Standard Protocol

TTT is performed under regional or general anesthesia with the patient in the supine position. A longitudinal curvilinear skin incision approximately 4 to 5 cm in length is made over the anteromedial proximal tibia, positioned 3 to 5 cm distal to the tibial tuberosity. Given the indications of this procedure, care should be taken when planning both the incision and pin placement to avoid compromising a possible future below-knee amputation. The periosteum is preserved—a critical step that ensures robust vascular supply to the transport fragment and maximizes the angiogenic response.[2,5] Using a series of 2.0 to 2.5 mm drill holes subsequently connected with a thin osteotome versus narrow oscilatting saw, a rectangular cortical bone window measuring approximately 5 × 1.5 cm is fashioned through the anteromedial cortex.[2,3] Cortical window placement relies on standard surgical landmarks and direct visualization; routine preoperative CT is not required for the standard procedure.[5,7]

Two half-pins are inserted into the corticotomized bone fragment; these should be placed prior to completion of the corticotomy to avoid premature detachment of the fragment. Two stabilizing half-pins are placed bicortically in the intact tibial shaft proximal and distal to the fragment, enabling assembly of a unilateral external fixator with a linking distraction device.[3] After a latency period of approximately 5-7 days, outward distraction is initiated at a rate of 1 mm per day for 10-14 days, achieving approximately 10-14 mm of lateral displacement. Following a 3 day consolidation rest at maximal displacement, reverse transport at the same rate over the subsequent 10-14 days returns the fragment to its anatomic position—the "accordion technique."[3,4] Two weeks after completion of transport, the external fixator is removed, for a total fixation duration of approximately 5 weeks. The bidirectional nature of this movement is believed to maximize angiogenic signaling by delivering repeated cycles of mechanical stimulation.[4]

Patients are typically permitted to bear weight during the fixation period, with heel offloading recommended when the wound involves the plantar hindfoot. Total operative time in experienced hands averages 35 to 45 minutes with minimal blood loss.

Modified Techniques and Technical Variations

Several modifications to the standard protocol have been described with favorable results. A dual-window approach using 2 smaller 1.5 × 1.5 cm^2 bone windows achieved a 95.83% healing rate in 98 patients with no tibial fractures, potentially reducing fracture risk by limiting the proportion of cortical circumference removed at any single level.[30] A combined bone-and-periosteum transfer modification—in which the periosteum is repaired after corticotomy and transported together—preserves periosteal vascularity and was associated with 93.75% healing and reduced osteonecrosis risk in 48 patients with Wagner grade 3 to 4 disease.[31] North American series have employed a slightly longer latency period of 10 days and slower distraction rate of 0.5 mm per day divided into 2 daily increments (0.25 mm each), reflecting adaptation to multimorbid patient populations including those with end-stage renal disease or active calcaneal osteomyelitis.[32–34] A minimally invasive percutaneous TTT approach using smaller incisions has also been described, maintaining the core biomechanical principles while reducing operative morbidity at the tibial site.[34]

Three Dimensional-printed and Technology-assisted Approaches

For surgeons seeking enhanced osteotomy precision or those early in their learning curve, customized 3 dimensional (3D)-printed osteotomy guide plates designed from preoperative CT data represent an optional technological adjunct. In a prospective evaluation of 17 patients, this approach showed no significant deviation from preoperative design parameters across 5 key bone window measurements, with a mean osteotomy duration of 35 ± 15 minutes and no intraoperative bone window fractures.[35] Complete bone window incorporation and full wound healing were confirmed at 4 to 8 months. These guides are not required for routine TTT but may reduce the learning curve in early-adopter settings or facilitate training.

Dedicated External Fixation Devices

The global expansion of TTT has been accompanied by development of purpose-built unilateral external fixation systems that standardize the technique and improve reproducibility. The Cybion TTT system (CE-marked, European Union) is based on a clinical dataset of more than 1200 cases and incorporates a precision transport screw with a corticotomy guide that preserves periosteal integrity.[20] The Orthofix TrueLok Elevate system achieved Food and Drug Administration (FDA) 510(k) clearance in 2025 as the first TTT-specific device approved in the United States, featuring 0.25 mm increment precision adjustments and a sterile corticotomy guide kit.[20] These dedicated systems substantially reduce the technical complexity of the procedure and lower the barrier to adoption by surgeons without prior Ilizarov experience.

BIOMECHANICAL CONSIDERATIONS

Finite element analysis using 3 D CT-derived tibial models has established the biomechanical safety of the standard TTT cortical window.[1,36] Creation of the 5 × 1.5 cm^2 window in the proximal tibial metaphysis does not significantly compromise overall structural integrity under physiologic loading, with stress concentrations primarily localized around half-pin insertion sites and the cortical window margins rather than distributed across the tibial diaphysis.[1] The external fixator provides substantial load sharing during the active transport phase, further mitigating fracture risk.

Fracture risk is greatest when the cortical window extends into the narrower middiaphyseal or distal tibial cortex, where the medullary canal is more constrained. Positioning the window within the broader proximal metaphysis, using standard anatomic landmarks and direct surgical visualization, minimizes this risk and is consistent with the approach described across the major published series.[5,7,36] These findings support the mechanical safety of the technique when standard postoperative weight-bearing restrictions are observed throughout the 5 week fixation period.

CLINICAL OUTCOMES

Wound Healing

The most comprehensive clinical evidence comes from the prospective multicenter cohort by Chen and colleagues[5] (CORR), which enrolled 249 consecutive patients with severe and recalcitrant DFUs and compared TTT directly against conventional surgical management including arterial reconstruction and flap transplants. The ulcer healing rate was 96% in the TTT group versus 72% with conventional treatment ($P<.001$), and limb salvage was 97.1% versus 77.4% ($P<.001$) at 2 year follow-up. A larger 7 center prospective cohort by the same group subsequently enrolled 1175 patients, confirming a 94.9% healing rate with a mean healing time of 12.4 ± 5.6 weeks, a major amputation rate of 4.9%, and a recurrence rate of only 3.1%.[1]

The meta-analysis by Hu and colleagues,[8] pooling 7 comparative studies involving 818 participants, provides the highest-level quantitative synthesis available. The pooled healing rate was 0.96 (95% confidence interval [95%CI]: 0.93–0.98) and the pooled limb salvage rate was 0.98 (95%CI: 0.95–1.00). Compared to non-TTT controls, TTT was associated with a healing OR of 10.43 (95%CI: 3.96–27.43, $P<.001$) and a limb salvage OR of 9.65 (95%CI: 3.30–28.20, $P<.001$). DFU recurrence was reduced by 82% in TTT-treated patients (RR 0.18, 95%CI: 0.06–0.49, $P = .001$). The Luxon and colleagues systematic review of 13 studies (924 patients) similarly identified a 26% point absolute difference in healing rates favoring TTT over conventional care.[2]

High healing and limb salvage rates have been confirmed across a range of special clinical scenarios. Among 21 patients with large diabetic heel ulcers (mean wound area 67 cm^2)—a notoriously difficult wound location—100% limb salvage and complete wound healing were achieved with a mean healing time of 128.6 days.[14,37] The first international case series from Singapore reported 100% limb salvage with a median healing time of 4 months, confirming the technique's reproducibility outside its country of origin.[7]

Vascular and Perfusion Outcomes

Objective vascular improvement is consistently documented across the literature. ABI improvements in the range of 0.2 to 0.4 points above preoperative baselines are typical, with a pooled ABI improvement of MD +0.23 reported in the Hu and colleagues[8] meta-analysis ($P<.001$). Multiple studies document ABI normalization from ischemic (<0.9) to near-normal (>0.8) ranges following TTT. Serial growth factor measurements in 19 Wagner stage 4 DFU patients showed significant elevations in VEGF, bFGF, and PDGF from day 11 onward, with digital subtraction angiography at 3 months confirming thickening of calf and foot arteries and a rich collateral vascular network.[38] Foot skin temperature improvements from approximately 33.4°C to 36.0°C further corroborate improved distal perfusion.

Pain Relief and Quality of Life

The Hu and colleagues[8] meta-analysis reported a pooled VAS pain improvement of MD 3.70 points (95%CI: 1.97–5.44, $P<.001$). In a 70 patient comparative study, TTT produced significantly lower VAS scores alongside superior ABI and neuropathy screening scores compared to conventional wound debridement ($P<.05$).[17] Quality of life assessed by SF-36 component scores was significantly improved at 2 year follow-up in the large multicenter cohort, underscoring TTT's functional as well as anatomic benefits.[1]

Nondiabetic and Expanded Indications

TTT's indications extend meaningfully beyond DFU. In a prospective comparative study of 85 patients with recalcitrant nondiabetic leg ulcers of arterial, venous, and mixed etiology, TTT achieved significantly higher 1 year healing rates (78.6% vs 58.1%, OR 2.64, $P = .04$) and shorter healing times (4.5 vs 6.1 months, $P = .02$) compared to conventional surgery, with CTA confirming increased small vessel density throughout the ipsilateral limb.[11] For thromboangiitis obliterans, a 119 patient retrospective study demonstrated TTT's superiority over conventional treatment across functional recovery, hemorheological parameters, and quality of life measures, with age, hepatitis B status, and treatment approach identified as independent prognostic factors.[12] TTT has also been applied to ischemic Charcot midfoot reconstruction: a case from King's College Hospital documented simultaneous lateral TTT and Charcot deformity correction in a patient refractory to multiple prior revascularization attempts, achieving bone fusion at 6 months with no complications at 27 month follow-up.[39]

COMBINATION WITH REVASCULARIZATION

The integration of TTT with EVT addresses both macrovascular and microvascular components of CLTI simultaneously. In a retrospective comparison of 131 patients, combined TTT plus EVT achieved amputation-free survival (AFS) of 85.5% at 6 months and 81.9% at 12 months, compared with 72.4% and 48.9%, respectively, for EVT alone.[3] At 24 months, 74.2% of the combined group remained amputation-free with all surviving patients achieving wound healing—a durability that suggests TTT's microvascular effects extend well beyond the period of active treatment.

The sequential approach of first optimizing macrovascular inflow with EVT, then applying TTT to drive microvascular proliferation, is recommended by the CAOS expert consensus.[19] The rationale is that restored macrovascular flow provides a richer substrate of circulating progenitors and growth factors for TTT to mobilize to the wound site. In patients unsuitable for revascularization, TTT alone can still achieve meaningful outcomes: in the Chen and colleagues[5] cohort, only 7.6% underwent revascularization yet 96% of ulcers healed, suggesting that TTT's microvascular effects may partially compensate for the absence of macrovascular intervention in selected patients.

In disease patterns characterized by diffuse small-vessel involvement—such as thromboangiitis obliterans—where endovascular targets are limited, TTT may be uniquely effective as a standalone treatment. Zuo and colleagues[15] demonstrated that TTT outperformed percutaneous transluminal balloon angioplasty across artery diameter, blood flow, wound healing time, pain resolution, and growth factor expression in patients with chronic lower limb ischemia.

COMPLICATIONS

The safety profile of TTT is generally favorable relative to the severity of the treated patient population. Pin-site infection is the most commonly reported complication, occurring in approximately 2.1% of patients in the largest cohort and a pooled risk of 0.08 in the Hu and colleagues meta-analysis.[1,8] Most infections respond to local wound care and oral antibiotics without requiring fixator removal. In several Western series, no pin-site infections were reported, suggesting that meticulous pin care protocols can minimize this risk further.[7,32,33]

Tibial fracture at the corticotomy site is the most serious procedural complication, with a pooled risk of 0.02 in the meta-analysis.[8] In the large multicenter cohort, 8 of 1072 patients (0.7%) sustained closed tibial fractures, all of which healed uneventfully with continued external fixation.[1] Intraoperative drill fractures have been reported when the osteotomy was positioned in the narrower middiaphyseal tibia,[3] underscoring the importance of accurate anatomic window placement using direct visualization and standard landmarks.

A prognostic factor analysis of 120 diabetic foot patients identified 4 independent predictors of adverse postoperative outcome: low foot skin temperature, low transcutaneous oxygen pressure ($TcPO_2$), elevated fasting blood glucose, and raised CRP—with a combined discriminatory AUC of 0.998.[13] These findings provide actionable preoperative risk stratification targets. Additional reported adverse events include superficial wound breakdown at the corticotomy incision site, transient edema and pain during the transport period, osteotomy margin necrosis (8.33% in Liu and colleagues), lower limb venous thrombosis (5.83%), and rare cases of mild cortical fragment displacement due to premature fixator removal. No reports of catastrophic tibial failure, permanent neurovascular injury, or procedure-related mortality attributable to TTT have been published in the reviewed literature.

INDICATIONS AND PATIENT SELECTION

Based on the CAOS expert consensus and the cumulative evidence reviewed, TTT is indicated in patients with severe DFUs of Texas University grade 2C to 3D, CLTI with ischemic ulceration refractory to conventional therapy, recalcitrant nondiabetic leg ulcers, lower limb thromboangiitis obliterans, and—in selected cases—ischemic Charcot neuroarthropathy requiring foot reconstruction.[11,12,19,39] The CAOS guidelines recommend TTT for wounds that have failed to respond to at least 4 to 8 weeks of appropriate management, with relative prerequisites including adequate proximal tibial anatomy, absence of active infection at the corticotomy site, wound location more than 5 cm from the planned osteotomy, and ability to tolerate external fixation for 5 weeks.[19]

Preoperative risk stratification is guided by the prognostic factor data from Liu and colleagues,[13] which identified $TcPO_2$, foot skin temperature, fasting blood glucose, and serum CRP as the 4 most discriminatory predictors of adverse outcomes. Optimization of glycemic control and active infection prior to TTT is critical. For patients with concurrent macrovascular disease amenable to endovascular correction, performing EVT before or concurrently with TTT may enhance outcomes by maximizing the vascular substrate available for TTT-driven microvascular proliferation.[3]

Bilateral DFUs represent a special indication. Qin and colleagues demonstrated that unilateral TTT produces systemic angiogenic effects sufficient to promote healing in both limbs, with comparable 1 year healing rates in bilateral and unilateral DFU patients (76.5% vs 91.2%, $P = .10$) confirmed by bilateral CTA neovascularization.[9,40] This finding suggests that a single TTT procedure may address bilateral disease, with substantial clinical and economic implications.

Contraindications include active malignancy within the wound, acute critical limb ischemia requiring emergency revascularization, active infection at the corticotomy site, inability to tolerate external fixation, severe systemic contraindications to surgery, and wounds extending within 5 cm of the planned osteotomy. Stable dialysis patients have been treated successfully in some series, though severe immunosuppression remains a relative contraindication in most published protocols.[19,32]

DISCUSSION

TTT represents a fundamental paradigm shift in the surgical management of ischemic lower extremity disease. Rather than attempting to correct macrovascular anatomy—which addresses only one component of a multifactorial pathophysiology—TTT leverages the body's endogenous regenerative capacity through mechanobiologic stimulation, triggering self-amplifying cascades of angiogenesis, immunomodulation, and tissue repair at the microcirculatory level. The breadth and consistency of beneficial outcomes across diverse clinical settings, patient populations, and disease etiologies—DFU, CLTI, thromboangiitis obliterans, nondiabetic leg ulcers, and Charcot reconstruction—suggest that TTT's effects are mediated by fundamental biologic mechanisms conserved across ischemic wound pathologies.

The molecular mechanistic landscape of TTT has been substantially clarified by the studies reviewed, revealing multiple overlapping pathways by which tibial microinjury translates into angiogenesis and wound healing at a remote site. These involve growth factor release, bone marrow-derived progenitor cell mobilization, immune cell polarization toward a reparative phenotype, and paracrine signaling through circulating vesicles and proteins. Importantly, this mechanistic diversity may explain both the robustness of TTT's clinical effects across different disease types and the potential for pharmacologic augmentation—as demonstrated by a clinical trial in which oral compounds that mimic aspects of TTT's molecular effects achieved meaningful acceleration of wound closure in patients with refractory DFUs.[25]

The evolution of TTT from improvised ring fixators to purpose-built, FDA-cleared unilateral systems marks a critical maturation toward standardization and global accessibility. The first international case series from Singapore[7] and regulatory clearances in the EU and United States[20] signal that TTT's geographic footprint is expanding beyond its Chinese origins. However, the vast majority of published evidence—including all large cohort studies and both systematic reviews—originates from Chinese institutions, raising important questions about generalizability to non-Asian populations with different comorbidity profiles, health care systems, and disease characteristics.

Significant limitations of the current evidence base must be acknowledged. The absence of randomized controlled trials is the most critical gap; most studies are retrospective single-center or multicenter cohorts with heterogeneous concomitant treatments, variable wound classification systems, and nonstandardized outcome reporting. The optimal distraction rate, latency period, window dimensions, and transport duration remain subjects of ongoing investigation. Future high-quality prospective randomized trials—comparing TTT plus standard care versus standard care alone, or TTT plus EVT versus EVT alone—using standardized wound classification and outcome measures are essential to definitively establish TTT's place in evidence-based limb salvage pathways.

Health economic analyses are also seriously needed. Although TTT involves upfront procedural cost and a 5 week external fixation period, the potential to avert major amputation—with its associated costs of prosthetics, rehabilitation, lost productivity, and markedly elevated long-term mortality—could render it highly cost-effective. The 82% reduction in DFU recurrence reported by Hu and colleagues[8] (RR 0.18, $P = .001$) further suggests that TTT's economic benefits extend well beyond the index hospitalization.

SUMMARY

TTT is an established adjunctive surgical technique for limb salvage in patients with severe ischemic lower extremity disease, supported by a growing evidence base encompassing more than 3000 patients across 35 publications. By targeting microvascular dysfunction through biologically driven angiogenesis and immunomodulation, TTT addresses a pathophysiologic dimension that macrovascular revascularization alone cannot adequately correct. The meta-analysis by Hu and colleagues reported pooled healing and limb salvage rates of 0.96 and 0.98, respectively, with dramatically superior outcomes versus non-TTT controls—consistent with the high rates reported across individual cohort studies reviewed here. These findings, alongside dramatic reductions in recurrence and meaningful quality-of-life improvements, are consistent across diverse patient populations and disease etiologies.

TTT complements rather than replaces conventional revascularization strategies, and the combination of TTT with EVT offers superior AFS in severe CLTI. Its indications now encompass nondiabetic leg ulcers, thromboangiitis obliterans, and ischemic Charcot reconstruction.

Complications are generally minor and manageable with proactive monitoring.

Further high-quality prospective randomized trials, standardized international protocols, and health economic analyses are required to consolidate TTT's role within evidence-based multidisciplinary limb salvage pathways. Integration of TTT into structured diabetic foot care teams—encompassing endocrinologists, vascular surgeons, orthopedic surgeons, wound care specialists, and podiatrists—is essential to optimize patient selection, surgical execution, and long-term outcomes.

CLINICS CARE POINTS

- Patient selection is paramount: optimize glycemic control, transcutaneous oxygen pressure, and CRP before TTT; patients with severely impaired tissue oxygenation ($TcPO_2$ <30 mm Hg) may require concurrent or staged revascularization to maximize response.
- Plan the incision and half-pin placement with a possible future below-knee amputation in mind; the TTT corticotomy site should not compromise standard amputation flaps or tibial bone stock required for prosthetic fitting.
- The cortical window should be positioned 3 to 5 cm distal to the tibial tuberosity using direct anatomic landmarks; routine preoperative CT is not required. Avoid the middiaphysis and distal tibia where medullary canal narrowing significantly increases fracture risk.
- While ideal guidelines on distraction protocol are in consideration, largely distraction should begin after a 5 day latency period at 1 mm per day for 10 days, followed by a 3 day rest, then reverse transport at the same rate—the "accordion technique"; significantly deviating from this protocol (eg, faster distraction) risks inadequate neovascularization or premature consolidation.
- Combining TTT with EVT produces significantly better AFS at 12 and 24 months than EVT alone in CLTI; when macrovascular disease is amenable to correction, EVT should be performed first or concurrently.
- Unilateral TTT can produce bilateral angiogenic effects; a single procedure may be sufficient to address bilateral DFUs, avoiding the morbidity of staged bilateral surgery.
- Pin-site infections, the most common complication, are largely preventable with standardized daily pin care protocols and early oral antibiotic treatment at the first sign of erythema or drainage.
- Dedicate ongoing postoperative wound care alongside TTT; in complex wounds, integration with debridement, negative-pressure wound therapy, and skin grafting further improves healing rates, as demonstrated in the integrated surgical wound treatment protocol.

During the preparation of this article, the authors used Gen AI. After using this tool/service, the authors reviewed and edited the content as needed and take full responsibility for the content of the publication.

DISCLOSURE

S. Raszka: nothing to disclose. M. Michalski: Consultant, Speaker-Arthrex | Consultant, IP Holder-Extremity Medical | Consultant-Paragon 28, C. Moon: Consultant-Stryker Trauma|Consultant-Corentec (Relationship has ended) | Consultant-Paragon28 (Relationship has ended) | Consultant-Globus Medical|Consultant-Acumed | Consultant-Extremity Medical | Consultant-SI Bone | Speaker-My01 | Speaker-Illuminoss | Speaker-Bone Support.

REFERENCES

1. Chen Y, Ding X, Zhu Y, et al. Effect of tibial cortex transverse transport in patients with recalcitrant diabetic foot ulcers: a prospective multicenter cohort study. J Orthop Transl 2022;36:194–204.
2. Luxon A, Syziu A, Harrison WD, et al. A systematic review on tibial cortex transverse transport in the treatment of ischemic ulcers of the lower limb. Foot Ankle Int 2025;46(8):914–24.
3. Ding Y, Yu D, Huang H, et al. Combining tibial cortex transverse transport and endovascular therapy for limb salvage in chronic limb-threatening ischemia. Orthop Surg 2024;16:2132–9.
4. Ilizarov GA. The tension-stress effect on the genesis and growth of tissues. Part I. Clin Orthop Relat Res 1989;238:249–81.
5. Chen Y, Kuang X, Zhou J, et al. Proximal tibial cortex transverse distraction facilitating healing and limb salvage in severe and recalcitrant diabetic foot ulcers. Clin Orthop Relat Res 2020;478(4):836–51.
6. Hua Q, Zhang Y, Wan C, et al. CAOS clinical guideline for TTT in diabetic foot ulcers (version 2020). J Orthop Transl 2020;25:11–6.
7. Wong JY, Sebastian M, Hua Q, et al. Transverse tibial transport: surgical technique and insights from first international case series. Int Wound J 2025;22:e70762.

8. Hu XX, Xiu ZZ, Li GC, et al. Effectiveness of transverse tibial bone transport in DFU: a systematic review and meta-analysis. Front Endocrinol 2023;13:1095361.
9. Qin W, Nie X, Su H, et al. Unilateral tibial cortex transverse transport on bilateral DFUs: propensity score matching study. J Orthop Transl 2023;42:137–46.
10. Liu J, Huang X, Su H, et al. Tibial cortex transverse transport facilitates severe diabetic foot wound healing via HIF-1α-induced angiogenesis. J Inflamm Res 2024;17:2681–96.
11. Nie X, Kuang X, Liu G, et al. Tibial cortex transverse transport facilitating healing in recalcitrant non-diabetic leg ulcers. J Orthop Transl 2021;27:1–7.
12. Hong M, Jin Q. Therapeutic effects of transverse tibial bone transport in lower limb thromboangiitis obliterans. Am J Transl Res 2025;17(6):4331–40.
13. Liu N, Dai S, Liu D, et al. Application of transverse tibial bone transfer in diabetic foot patients: prognostic and risk factors. Orthop Surg 2025;17:2708–16.
14. Jianda X, Maosheng B, et al. Novel treatment for large heel ulceration in diabetic patients: proximal tibial cortex transverse distraction. Int Wound J 2023;20:732–9.
15. Zuo Q, Gao F, Song H, et al. Ilizarov transverse tibial bone transport in chronic ischemic lower limb diseases. Exp Ther Med 2018;16:1355–9.
16. Chang S, Zhang F, Chen W, et al. Outcomes of integrated surgical wound treatment based on tibial transverse transport. Front Surg 2023;9:1051366.
17. Wen R, Cheng X, Cao H, et al. Transverse tibial bone transfer in the treatment of diabetes foot ulcer: a pilot study. Diabetes Metab Syndr Obes 2023;16:2005–12.
18. Qu L, Wang A, Tang F. The therapy of transverse tibial bone transport and vessel regeneration operation on thromboangitis obliterans. Zhonghua Yixue Zazhi 2001;81(10):622–4.
19. Hua Q, Zhang Y, Wan C, et al. CAOS clinical guideline for TTT technique (version 2020). J Orthop Transl 2020;25:11–6.
20. Transverse Tibial Cortex Transport (TTCT): Latest devices, techniques, and future directions. [Project file: TTCT review, 2025.] Orthofix TrueLok Elevate FDA 510(k) clearance 2025; Cybion CE-mark .
21. Ou S, Wu X, Yang Y, et al. Tibial cortex transverse transport potentiates diabetic wound healing via activation of SDF-1/CXCR4 signaling. PeerJ 2023;11:e15894.
22. Tian W, Zhang L, Wang Y, et al. Tibial transverse transport promotes wound healing in DFUs by stimulating EPC mobilization and homing. Ann Med 2024;56(1):2404186.
23. Yang Y, Li Y, Pan Q, et al. Tibial cortex transverse transport accelerates wound healing via enhanced angiogenesis and immunomodulation. Bone Joint Res 2022;11(4):189–99.
24. Yu L, Zhang D, Yin Y, et al. Tibial cortex transverse transport surgery improves wound healing in severe type 2 DFUs by activating a systemic immune response. Int J Surgery 2025;111:257–72.
25. Xie J, Liu X, Wu B, et al. Bone transport induces the release of factors with multi-tissue regenerative potential for diabetic wound healing. Cell Rep Med 2024;5:101588.
26. Huang X, Liu J, Wu X, et al. Remote continuous microinjury-triggered cytokines facilitate severe DFU healing via the Ras/Raf/MEK/ERK pathway. J Inflamm Res 2025;18:1755–72.
27. Kong L, Li Y, Deng Z, et al. Tibial cortex transverse transport regulates Orai1/STIM1-mediated NO release and improves vessel migration via osteopontin. J Orthop Transl 2024;45:107–19.
28. Su H, Zhen P, Hou J, et al. Finite element analysis of tibial cortex transverse transport. Bone Joint Res 2025;14:281–91.
29. Qin W, Liu K, Su H, et al. Tibial cortex transverse transport promotes ischemic DFU healing via enhanced angiogenesis in a novel rat model. Eur J Med Res 2024;29:155.
30. Liu J, Yao X, Xu Z, et al. Modified tibial cortex transverse transport for DFUs with Wagner grade ≥II: 98 patients. Front Endocrinol 2024;15:1334414.
31. Wen Y, Chen LY, Lan JP, et al. Management of severe diabetic foot using modified transverse bone transport: wagner grade 3–4 cases. Medicine 2025;104:49. e45387.
32. Yang AA, Park N, Gazes MI, et al. Transverse tibial bone transport for non-healing heel wound: case report. Int J Surg Case Rep 2024;124:110400.
33. Estes A, Samchukov M. Transverse tibial bone transport to avoid major lower limb amputation: case report. Int J Surg Case Rep 2025;133:111508.
34. Li G, Ling SKK, Li HA, et al. Minimally invasive tibial cortex transverse transport surgery. J Orthop Transl 2020;25:28–32.
35. Wei D, Zhou W, Huang J, et al. Application of a customized 3D-printed osteotomy guide plate for tibial transverse transport. Sci Rep 2024;14:22771.
36. Zhen P, Liu J, Su H, et al. Finite element analysis of biomechanical effects during tibial cortex transverse transport. [Project file: Finite_element_analysis.pdf].
37. Mukherjee S, Im SS. Impact of tibial transverse transport in tissue regeneration and wound healing with perspective on DFUs. World J Diabetes 2024; 15(5):810–3.
38. Ou S, Xu C, Yang Y, et al. Transverse tibial bone transport enhances distraction osteogenesis and vascularization in diabetic foot. Orthop Surg 2022;14:2170–9.
39. Al Omar H, Lahoti O, Edmonds M, et al. Ischaemic Charcot midfoot reconstruction combined with lateral tibial cortex transverse transport: case report. Strategies Trauma Limb Reconstr 2025;20(1):50–5.
40. Zhang X, Dong T, Yao S, et al. Application of transverse tibial bone transport in DFU: case report. Ann Palliat Med 2021;10(7):8358–64.

Pediatrics

Pediatric Regenerative Medicine

A Focus on Distraction Osteogenesis

Alyssa Barré, MD[a], Dylan Kluck, MD[a,b,*]

KEYWORDS

• Bone regeneration • Distraction osteogenesis • Limb lengthening • Pediatric orthopedics
• Regenerative medicine • Regenerate salvage

KEY POINTS

- Distraction osteogenesis represents a model of regenerative medicine in pediatric orthopedics, integrating mechanics and biology.
- Successful regenerate formation depends on meticulous perioperative planning, appropriate distraction parameters, and preservation of the biologic environment.
- When regenerate quality is compromised, a spectrum of mechanical, biophysical, and biologic strategies may be employed to optimize or salvage bone formation.

INTRODUCTION

Regenerative medicine is a field that aims to repair, replace, or augment tissues or organs to restore function through a variety of approaches including tissue engineering, immunotherapy, biologics, and stem cell therapy. The field of regenerative medicine in pediatric orthopedics represents a unique interface where advanced biologic strategies are applied to a population with significant regenerative potential. Complementing the metabolic and remodeling capacity inherent to the physis and periosteum, the pediatric skeleton, therefore, represents an intriguing target for regenerative medicine.

The application of regenerative medicine within pediatric orthopedics is broad. For example, percutaneous injection of bone marrow aspirate concentrate (BMAC) combined with demineralized bone matrix can help avoid open surgery for unicameral bone cysts[1]; allograft, bone morphogenetic protein (BMP), and bioactive glass can be used to enhance arthrodesis for scoliosis[2,3]; the field of pediatric sports medicine is rich in applications of platelet-rich plasma, autografts and allografts, and cartilage restoration/transplantation procedures[4–6]; and gene therapy for conditions such as Duchenne muscular dystrophy, osteogenesis imperfecta, and spinal muscular atrophy has been a relatively recent but promising effort.[7] However, one of the most profound applications of regenerative medicine principles in this population, and the primary focus of this review, is distraction osteogenesis (DO), a process of functional tissue engineering that utilizes the body's innate biologic response to mechanical stimuli to create native, vascularized bone and soft tissue. This review synthesizes the biologic principles underlying DO, perioperative factors influencing regenerate quality, and mechanical, biophysical, and biologic salvage strategies for compromised regenerate in pediatric limb lengthening.

[a] Department of Orthopaedic Surgery and Sports Medicine, University of Kentucky, Lexington, KY, USA; [b] Department of Orthopaedic Surgery, Shriners Children's Lexington, Lexington, KY, USA
* Corresponding author. Department of Orthopaedic Surgery, Shriners Children's Lexington, 110 Conn Terrace, Lexington, KY 40508.
E-mail address: dylan.kluck@shrinenet.org

Orthop Clin N Am 57 (2026) 349–358
https://doi.org/10.1016/j.ocl.2026.05.008

Abbreviations	
BMAC	bone marrow aspirate concentrate
BMP	bone morphogenetic protein
DO	distraction osteogenesis
ESWT	extracorporeal shock wave therapy
HBO	hyperbaric oxygen therapy
HIF-1α	hypoxia inducible factor 1-alpha
PRP	platelet-rich plasma
PVRs	pixel value ratios
VEGF	vascular endothelial growth factor

BIOLOGY AND PRINCIPLES OF BONE REGENERATION

Mechanotransduction and the Law of Tension Stress

The foundational mechanism of DO is the law of tension-stress, described by Gavriil Ilizarov, which dictates that gradual traction on living tissues stimulates and maintains the regeneration of those tissues. This occurs through mechanotransduction, where mechanical forces are converted into biochemical signals that activate cellular proliferation and biosynthetic functions.[8] At the molecular level, tension regulates a vast cluster of genes, including proto-oncogenes such as *c-fos* and *c-jun*, and signaling pathways such as Wnt and focal adhesion kinase, which direct stem cells toward an osteogenic pathway while the tissues are being distracted, and ceases once distraction halts.[8,9]

Angiogenesis and the Hypoxic Response

Vascular formation is the critical, rate-limiting step in successful bone regeneration.[10,11] DO is a highly vascular-dependent process where blood flow in the distraction gap can peak at up to 10 times control values during distraction at the osteotomy, persists at 3 times that of control for several months, and induces increase in blood flow distant to the regenerate.[12,13] This neovascularization is driven by tissue hypoxia, which stabilizes hypoxia inducible factor 1-alpha (HIF-1α). HIF-1α then promotes the expression of vascular endothelial growth factor (VEGF), ensuring a tight coupling between angiogenesis and osteogenesis.[14] Recent studies have refined our understanding of this process, showing that vascular development occurs by sequential intramuscular arteriogenesis (enlargement of existing vessels in the muscle) followed by intraosteal angiogenesis (formation of new small vessels within the bone) once distraction ceases.[10]

Muscle Adaptation During Distraction

Distraction histogenesis is the simultaneous, parallel generation of new soft tissues including muscles, nerves, vessels, and skin that keep in pace with osseous lengthening of DO.[15] Muscles lying parallel to the distraction vector undergo growth via both hypertrophy and hyperplasia, where new myocytes and sarcomeres are formed to accommodate the increased length.[15,16] Studies in animal models demonstrate that during modest lengthening (up to 10% of original length), the muscle adapts through a sliding effect and tighter packing of fibers.[17] However, as the magnitude of lengthening approaches and exceeds 20% of the bone's original length, the risk of pathologic adaptation increases.[17,18] Beyond this threshold, muscle and fascia often fail to maintain regenerative pace, leading to fibrosis, muscular degeneration, and joint contractures.[16,18]

Nerve Growth and Injury During Distraction

Nerves are arguably the most sensitive structures during distraction, and their response to tension is a major source of postoperative morbidity. During active distraction, the development of nerves progresses through axonogenesis to keep pace with the lengthening tissues. Tension stress causes upregulation of neurotrophins and their receptors, which are essential for survival and differentiation of neuronal cells.[19] However, when mechanical strain exceeds the capacity of the nerve to elongate, peripheral neuropathy ensues, manifesting clinically as paresthesias and numbness. If the tension is not relieved, the sensory disturbances can progress to motor loss or permanent paralysis.[15] The peroneal nerve is particularly vulnerable in lower extremity lengthening or deformity corrections.[20] Distraction rates, discussed in more detail later, exceeding 2.0 mm per day are consistently associated with neuropathies and denervation.[21] Any evidence of delayed-onset nerve deficits during lengthening requires an immediate response of slowing, stopping, or even reversing the lengthening to allow the nerve to recover from the traction injury.

PERIOPERATIVE FACTORS, TECHNIQUES, AND OPTIMIZATION

Preoperative Factors and Optimization

The success of DO is rooted in both meticulous preoperative surgical planning and preoperative optimization of the host's biological environment. While preoperative deformity analysis is outside the scope of this article, the rate of bone regeneration during distraction mimics fetal growth and, thus, the metabolic demands on the pediatric patient are significant.[22]

Before initiating DO, potential nutritional deficiencies that could impair osteogenesis should be addressed. It is recommended to check serum mineral levels and target a level of 25-OH Vitamin D between 75 and 150 nmol/L.[23] Animal models utilizing total enteral nutrition demonstrated that high-quality nutritional intake not only prevents weight loss associated with the stress of DO, but also doubles the volume of mineralized bone formed during the distraction phase.[22] Calcium and phosphate availability should be maintained, as these ions serve as the fundamental building blocks for the rapid mineralization required during the consolidation period.

Intraoperative Factors and Techniques

The intraoperative techniques employed directly influence the biologic environment in which distraction occurs and may predispose to regenerate failure if principles are violated.

Intramedullary versus external fixation regenerate

The mechanism of bone formation during DO (intramembranous vs endochondral vs transchondroid) is debated and likely a combination of pathways.[8] The pathways result in a regenerate that is biologically different when obtained by intramedullary lengthening nails compared to external frames, described by Bafor and colleagues.[24] Reaming for insertion of a lengthening nail strips the endosteal blood supply, and thus, the periosteal blood supply is the primary source of healing the regenerate. Intramedullary nails also limit axial micromotion more so than circular external frames. Additionally, while both intramedullary and external fixation distraction methods produce a "fibrous interzone" in the center of the regenerate, which converts to bone, intramedullary techniques form an additional "fibrous innerzone" circumferentially around the nail, which also converts to bone.[24] The result is that lengthening nail regenerate heals from the periphery to the center, as well as from the bone ends toward the center of the regenerate, and progressively thickens with time.[24] Another study that compared tibial lengthenings with and without nails found that lengthening with a nail results in more cylindrical and homogenous callus with better pixel value ratios (PVRs) and Ru Li classification.[25] An example of healing with a fibrous interzone in a patient with a circular frame is seen in Fig. 1A, contrasted with the patient healing through both fibrous interzone and innerzones with an intramedullary nail in Fig. 1B.

Low-energy corticotomy principles

The biological goal is to perform a minimally traumatic osteotomy that preserves the periosteum, endosteum, and bone marrow blood supply. Placement in the metaphysis is often preferred over the diaphysis because metaphyseal bone is rich in cancellous bone and has a superior blood supply, leading to more robust osteogenesis.[15,26] It is recommended to avoid high-speed power saws, as thermal necrosis of the bone ends is a common iatrogenic cause of delayed union and nonunion.[15,27]

Comparison of corticotomy techniques

1. Multiple drill hole osteotomy (De Bastiani Technique): This technique involves creating a series of percutaneous holes connected by an osteotome. The periosteum is preserved. This is the most commonly practiced pediatric technique, with a straightforward learning curve and reliable healing results. The bone shavings created by the drill act as an internal graft, releasing growth factors such as BMPs to induce local proliferation.[27]
2. Percutaneous Gigli saw (Afghan technique): This is a technique that provides a precise, clean cut after the Gigli saw is tunneled subperiosteally. There is minimal disruption to the periosteum or risk of thermal necrosis. Comparative studies have showed its biological superiority in tibial lengthening, with a significantly better healing index than the drill hole method (1.2 mo/cm versus 1.67 mo/cm. It does pose a risk of injury to surrounding soft tissues.[27,28]
3. Ilizarov corticotomy: This traditional method relies on corticotomy of two-thirds of the circumference of the cortex, finished by rotation of proximal and distal segments in opposite directions. While aimed at medullary preservation, it is the least precise method and carries a risk of unfavorable fracture propagation.[15,27]

Intraoperative orthobiologics and adjuncts

BMAC provides a source of concentrated mesenchymal stem cells, with 6-to-7 fold increase in nucleated cells compared to raw aspirate; platelet-rich plasma (PRP) provides osteoinductive growth factors such as VEGF and platelet-derived growth factor (PDGF), which enhance angiogenesis and mitogenesis in bone-forming cells.[29] In a randomized clinical

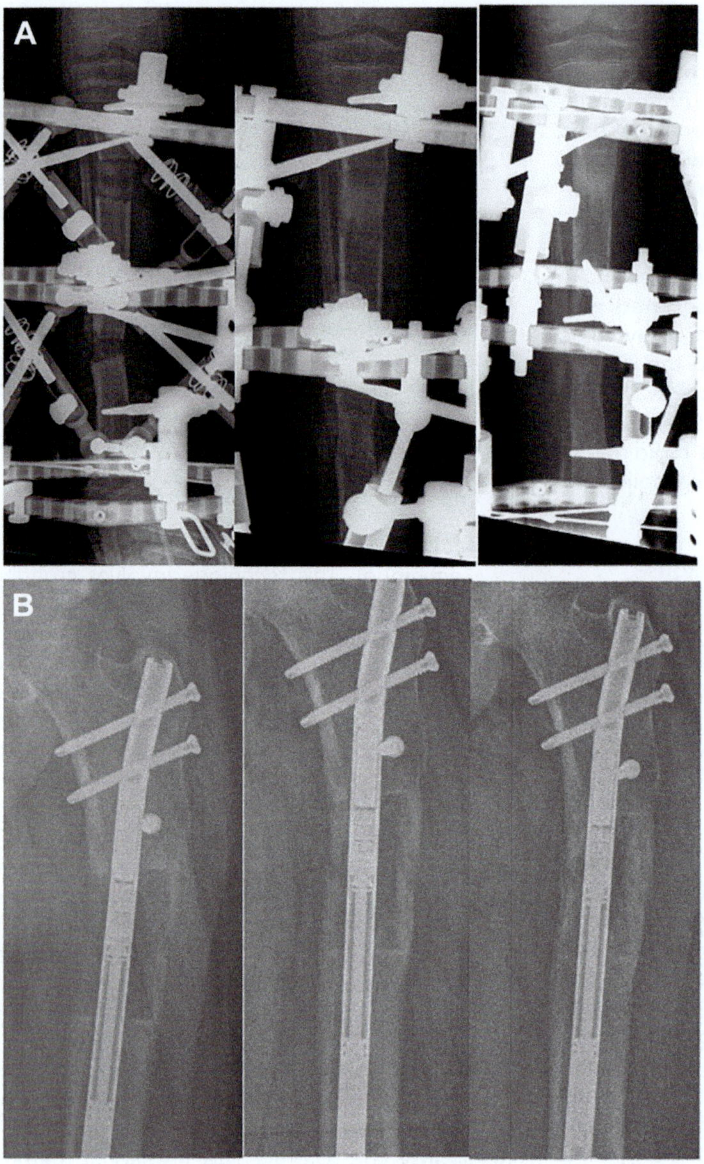

Fig. 1. (*A*) Patient with 2 level tibial corticotomies and circular frame with radiographic evidence of healing over time through the fibrous interzone. (*B*) Patient with femoral osteotomy and lengthening nail with radiographic evidence of healing over time through both the fibrous interzone and fibrous innerzone.

trial by Lee and colleagues,[29] patients received a combined injection of autologous BMAC and PRP at the tibial osteotomy site as the final step of the index surgery, utilizing 3 mL of BMAC combined with 3 mL of PRP for each segment that were obtained from the anterior superior iliac spine. This strategy resulted in significantly faster cortical healing indices across all 4 cortices. Further, the treatment group was permitted to fully weight-bear significantly earlier than the control group (0.99 vs 1.38 mo/cm), which was allowed once healing was observed at 2 cortices. Notably, these findings apply to augmentation at the index procedure and are separate from biologics that may be used for postoperative salvage, discussed later.

Postoperative Management of Distraction Osteogenesis

The postoperative management of DO is a meticulous process categorized into the latency, distraction, and consolidation phases, each relying on adequate mechanical and biological environments.

Rate and rhythm of distraction

A latency period of 3 to 10 days, varying based on patient age and quality of bone and soft tissue, occurs after the osteotomy and is intended to allow for the organization of reparative hematoma.[30] After the latency period, active distraction is initiated. The most commonly accepted distraction rate, based on the original teachings of Gavriil Ilizarov, is 1.0 mm per day, classically divided into a rhythm of 0.25 mm every 6 hours.[30,31] During the course of lengthening, however, the rate of lengthening may need to be adjusted based on radiographic assessment of regenerate, patient tolerance, and complications.[32] Importantly, a rate slower than 0.5 mm per day may lead to premature consolidation, effectively halting the procedure, while a rate exceeding 2 mm per day may lead to an atrophic, poor-quality regenerate with intertwined fibrous tissue and local ischemia.[8,15] Further, the rhythm of distraction influences bone quality, and newer automated distractors that provide continuous distraction have been shown to be biologically superior to manual increments with accelerated bone formation.[33] That said, there is no conclusive evidence that they offer better clinical outcomes or radiographic outcomes for long bone distraction and their additional cost may be unnecessary in children with robust bone-forming potential.[15,34]

Physiologic weight-bearing

Physiologic weight-bearing serves as a vital mechanical stimulus that is considered essential to the development and consolidation of newly formed bone in the distraction gap.[17] Mechanical loading stimulates intramembranous ossification and serves to minimize the loss of bone mineral in the native segments being lengthened, which helps prevent disuse osteopenia.[35] At the microvascular level, weight-bearing has been shown to increase both the number and length of newly formed vessels within the regenerate, facilitating matrix accumulation and modulating the local inflammatory response.[35] This loading provides beneficial axial micromotion that prevents stress shielding of the regenerate and assists in the transformation of the fibrous interzone into mineralized bone.[17] When utilizing external fixators, weight-bearing as tolerated is frequently encouraged to begin as early as the first postoperative day to allow for beneficial axial micromotion.[17] For patients undergoing intramedullary lengthening, the PVR—a metric that compares the density of the new bone in the distraction gap to the density of the adjacent native bone—can be utilized to determine when the regenerate has achieved sufficient density to safely advance to full weight-bearing.[36] In their study, Bafor and colleagues[36] determined that it was safe to progress to full weight-bearing once 3 of 4 cortices had a PVR of at least 0.92. Ultimately, the ability to bear weight earlier allows for a faster return to normal daily activities and may mitigate physiologic complications or physical debility associated with prolonged nonweight-bearing.

Mechanical and Biological Regenerate Optimization and Salvage Strategies

Despite meticulous surgical technique and adherence to distraction protocols, regenerate quality may still be compromised due to patient-specific, mechanical, or biological factors. Especially in pediatrics, bone disorders such as osteogenesis imperfecta or Rickets are often coexisting with the limb reconstruction. For a failing regenerate, surgical salvage with methods such as bone grafting or transition to a rigid nail are commonplace. However, there are additional salvage options that play into the regenerative properties of bone. Despite increasing clinical adoption, many of these regenerate optimization and salvage options either are supported predominantly by preclinical animal studies and small case series, with lack of large, prospective human studies or are extrapolated from adult literature.

Modulation of distraction rate and rhythm

The primary method for addressing a failing or suboptimal regenerative involves the case-dependent adjustment of the distraction protocol based on serial radiographic follow-up. If plain radiographs reveal a poor-quality regenerate, evidenced by multiple radiolucencies, an "hour-glass" configuration, or a delay in the appearance of bone formation beyond 30 days, the distraction rate should be slowed below the standard 1.0 mm per day. Some patients, especially in pediatric patients or those with pathologies such as Ollier's disease where bone formation is paradoxically accelerated,[37] distraction rates may need to be increased to prevent premature bridging of the distraction gap, which would otherwise necessitate a repeat surgical osteotomy.

Axial dynamization and preremoval optimization

Traditional axial dynamization is a mechanical strategy where a construct begins with rigid fixation and is subsequently converted to lower stiffness fixation as the healing process progresses. The primary objective of this approach is to gradually transfer physiologic loads from the hardware to the bone, thereby stimulating callus maturation and improving mechanical competence during the consolidation phase.[38] In clinical practice, this is often achieved by unlocking telescoping components, addition of in-line dynamization units, loosening the nuts on connection rods, or

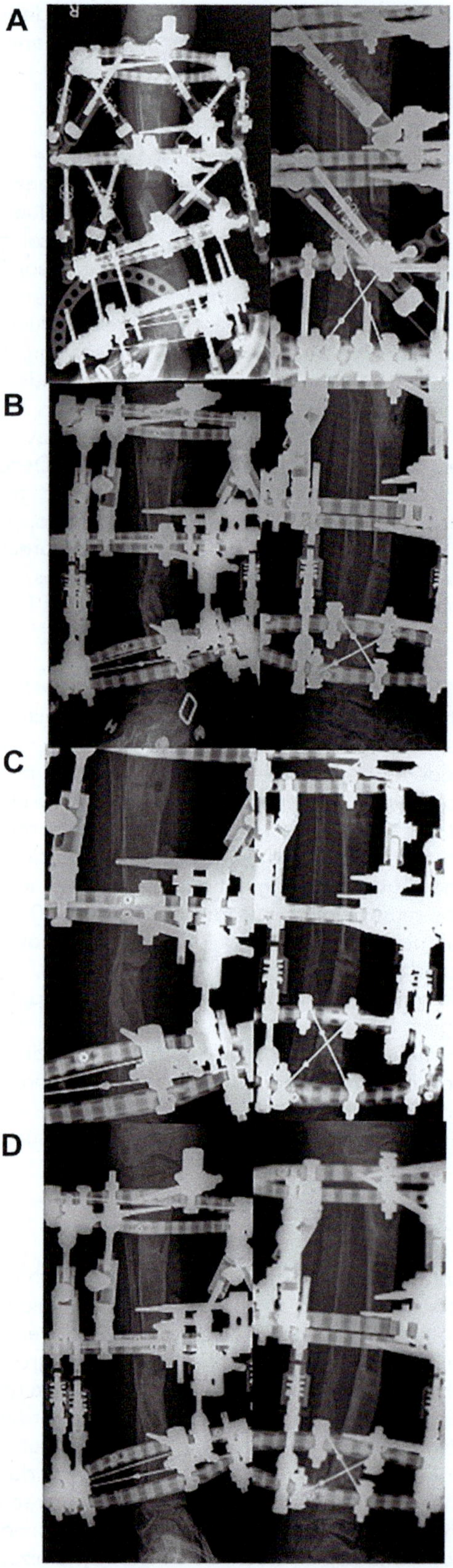

removing wires to allow for controlled axial movement while maintaining alignment. This technique is frequently employed as a preremoval optimization to ensure the bone regenerate is mechanically sufficient before the external fixator is removed.[39] A clinical example of this is shown in Fig. 2A–D, where a delayed regenerate was revived with addition of in-line dynamization units, and the regenerate then consolidated.

Optimization of construct stiffness through reverse dynamization of a frame

Maturation of the regenerate can be stimulated by applying the principles of reverse dynamization, which involves changing the fixator's stiffness to match the biologic phase of healing.[38] Evidence from animal models suggests that using flexible fixation to allow approximately 2 mm of axial micromotion during the active distraction phase promotes more abundant initial callus formation. Once the distraction is complete and the consolidation phase begins, the construct is converted to rigid fixation to prevent the disruption of newly formed vascularity during the final stages of remodeling. This transition results in a regenerate with higher bone mineral density and significantly greater torsional strength compared to maintaining a static or purely dynamic environment throughout the lengthening process.[38]

Mechanical manipulation via the accordion maneuver

When a regenerate appears atrophic or is failing to consolidate, the accordion maneuver, or cyclic distraction-compression, serves as a powerful but noninvasive salvage technique. This maneuver involves alternating periods of compression and distraction, typically in small incremental adjustments (eg, 0.25 mm per adjustment) applied over several days to weeks, to manipulate the mechanical environment of the distraction gap. Protocols vary across studies and may even differ by the issue (nonunion type vs hyporegenerate), but most emphasize modest daily magnitudes, maintenance of the original net lengthening goal, and close radiological surveillance to guide continuation or cessation as regenerate density and continuity improve.[40,41] Employing this strategy has been

Fig. 2. (*A*) Radiographs of a poorly healing distal tibial corticotomy after circular frame; (*B*) addition of in-line dynamization units to frame; (*C*) interval improvement in the radiographic appearance of the distal tibial regenerate; and (*D*) consolidation of the distal tibial regenerate.

described both during the distraction phase and early consolidation, and is frequently used as a first-line salvage technique. In a pooled clinical series of 80 patients treated with distraction-compression maneuvers in conjunction with Ilizarov reconstruction, a high bone healing rate and predominantly good/excellent functional outcomes were reported, with most patients achieving union following accordion technique application.[42] Biologically, these cyclic forces induce transient tissue hypoxia at the center of the distraction gap, which stabilizes hypoxia-inducible factor (HIF-1α) and subsequently upregulates VEGF. This process reboots the angiogenic-osteogenic coupling necessary for mineralization.[11,41]

Biophysical salvage: low-intensity pulsed ultrasound, pulsed electromagnetic fields, and extracorporeal shock wave therapy

Exogenous biophysical stimuli are established noninvasive salvage tools for delayed unions and suboptimal regenerates in both adult and pediatric patients. Low-intensity pulsed ultrasound delivers high-frequency acoustic pressure waves to the distraction site for 20 minutes daily, which upregulates proangiogenic factors and increases local blood flow. Clinical studies have shown it can reduce treatment time with minimal side effects.[43–45] Similarly, while off-label in children and with less conclusive evidence, pulsed electromagnetic fields has been shown to reduce bone loss distal to the distraction site, increase bone thickness and density, and allow for earlier fixator removal.[30,46,47] Extracorporeal shock wave therapy (ESWT) is an emerging biophysical modality that uses high-energy sound waves to stimulate bone regeneration by upregulating key angiogenic and osteogenic markers, including VEGF, bone morphogenetic protein-2 (BMP-2), and proliferating cell nuclear antigen (PCNA). Animal models show that ESWT improves mechanical bone strength, increases bone mineral density, and accelerates entry into the remodeling phase.[48] While results in animal limb and mandibular lengthening are promising, the specific effects and optimal dosing of ESWT in human pediatric populations have not yet been elucidated.[35]

Delayed orthobiologic injection

In cases where regenerate remains insufficient, biological adjuncts can be injected directly into the distraction gap. Transplantation of culture-expanded bone marrow cells combined with PRP into the distracted callus has been shown to accelerate osteogenesis, shorten the treatment period, and lower complications.[49] In contrast, evidence supporting delayed percutaneous BMAC injection for a failing regenerate remains sparse.

Systemic pharmacologic therapy

Systemic medications can be employed off-label to addresses specific deficiencies in the regenerate during the consolidation phase. Bisphosphonates, such as zoledronic acid or pamidronate, act as anticatabolic agents by inhibiting osteoclast-mediated resorption, thereby increasing the volume and mechanical strength of a failing catabolic regenerate and preventing disuse osteopenia.[23] In one small series, 6 of 7 children with failing regenerates were healed by systemic bisphosphates without the need for surgery and no systemic complications.[50]

Conversely, for an anabolic-insufficient regenerate, intermittent low-dose parathyroid hormone stimulates osteoblast activity and may promote osteogenesis.[51] However, its use is not well-established in DO, and it remains contraindicated in children and adolescents with open physes due to theoretic risk of osteosarcoma.[23]

Hyperbaric oxygen therapy

Hyperbaric oxygen therapy (HBO) is a salvage strategy that aims to promote bone maturation by maintaining high oxygen tension at the distraction site to counteract the regional hypoxia often found in failing regenerates. Biologically, HBO reduces endothelial damage by decreasing the ability of neutrophils to adhere to vessel walls, assists in restoring collagen production and fibroblast growth, replenishes stores of ATP, and limits local inflammatory response.[35] Experimental evidence suggests HBO can significantly accelerate both ossification and vascularization in the distraction gap, leading to increased bone mineral density.[52] Beyond its impact on osteogenesis, HBO helps mitigate the adverse effects of mechanical stretching on the surrounding skeletal muscle, promoting recovery in postischemic tissue and preserving contractile capacity by increasing muscle fibers and antioxidants.[53] While these findings indicate HBO can increase bone quality and quantity while shortening the consolidation period, its use as a standard salvage protocol in human DO is currently limited by a lack of extensive clinical trials.

SUMMARY

DO represents one of the most compelling clinical applications of regenerative medicine in pediatric orthopedics, integrating mechanical forces, vascular biology, and tissue adaptation to generate native bone and soft tissue. While meticulous surgical technique and adherence to established principles remain central to success, regenerate insufficiency may still arise, particularly in children with complex deformities or underlying metabolic or genetic bone conditions. A broad spectrum of mechanical, biophysical, and biologic strategies have therefore emerged to optimize or salvage compromised regenerate, reflecting an expanding understanding of how the biologic environment can be modulated throughout the lengthening process. Although the strength of supporting evidence varies across these interventions, their collective use illustrates how DO continues to serve as a dynamic model of regenerative medicine in practice and evolves alongside advances in biologic and biomechanical science.

CLINICS CARE POINTS

- Optimize host biology prior to DO by addressing nutritional deficiencies, vitamin D status, and underlying metabolic conditions.
- Adhere to biologically favorable surgical principles, including low-energy corticotomy techniques and thoughtful device selection.
- Maintain a low threshold to adjust the rate of distraction based on serial radiographic assessment of regenerate quality.
- At the earliest signs of suboptimal regenerate formation, consider mechanical, biophysical, or biologic rescue strategies.

DECLARATION OF GENERATIVE ARTIFICIAL INTELLIGENCE AND ARTIFICIAL INTELLIGENCE-ASSISTED TECHNOLOGIES IN THE WRITING PROCESS

AI (Grammarly) was used for syntax and language editing but source selection, interpretation, and synthesis were performed by the authors.

DISCLOSURE

The authors report no conflicts of interest related to this study.

REFERENCES

1. Gundle KR, Bhatt EM, Punt SE, et al. Injection of unicameral bone cysts with bone marrow aspirate and demineralized bone matrix avoids open curettage and bone grafting in a retrospective cohort. Open Orthop J 2017;11:486–92.
2. Letchuman V, Ampie L, Choy W, et al. Bone grafting and biologics for spinal fusion in the pediatric population: current understanding and future perspective. Neurosurg Focus 2021;50(6):E8.
3. Molinari RW, Kerr C, Kerr D. Bone morphogenetic protein in pediatric spine fusion surgery. J Spine Surg 2016;2(1):9–12.
4. Bray CC, Walker CM, Spence DD. Orthobiologics in pediatric sports medicine. Orthop Clin North Am 2017;48(3):333–42.
5. Syed AN, Landrum K, Ganley TJ. Platelet-rich plasma and other injectables in the young athlete. J Pediatr Soc North Am 2024;6:100008.
6. Otsuki S, Ikeda K, Tanaka K, et al. Implantation of novel meniscus scaffold for irreparable meniscal tear. Arthrosc Tech 2022;11(5):e775–9.
7. Olaonipekun E, Lisyansky A, Olaonipekun R, et al. Gene therapy in pediatric orthopedics. Osteology 2024;4(1).
8. Hamdy R, Rendon S, Tabrizian M. Distraction osteogenesis and its challenges in bone regeneration. In: Tal H, editor. Bone Regeneration. 2012. p. 185–212.
9. Kong L-C, Li HA, Kang Q-L, et al. An update to the advances in understanding distraction histogenesis: from biological mechanisms to novel clinical applications. J Orthop Transl 2020;25:3–10.
10. Morgan EF, Hussein AI, Al-Awadhi BA, et al. Vascular development during distraction osteogenesis proceeds by sequential intramuscular arteriogenesis followed by intraosteal angiogenesis. Bone 2012;51(3):535–45.
11. Liu Y, Cai F, Liu K, et al. Cyclic distraction-compression dynamization technique enhances the bone formation during distraction osteogenesis. Front Bioeng Biotechnol 2021;9:810723.
12. Aronson J. Temporal and spatial increases in blood flow during distraction osteogenesis. Clin Orthop Relat Res 1994;301:124–31.
13. Choi IH, Chung CY, Cho TJ, et al. Angiogenesis and mineralization during distraction osteogenesis. J Kor Med Sci 2002;17(4):435–47.
14. Wan C, Gilbert SR, Wang Y, et al. Activation of the hypoxia-inducible factor-1alpha pathway accelerates bone regeneration. Proc Natl Acad Sci U S A 2008;105(2):686–91.
15. Murray JH, Fitch RD. Distraction histiogenesis: principles and indications. J Am Acad Orthop Surg 1996;4(6):317–27.
16. Lindsey CA, Makarov MR, Shoemaker S, et al. The effect of the amount of limb lengthening on skeletal muscle. Clin Orthop Relat Res 2002;402:278–87.
17. Paley D. Current techniques of limb lengthening. J Pediatr Orthop 1988;8(1):73–92.

18. Adejuyigbe B, Gharpure M, Wahle CF, et al. Distraction osteogenesis: a comprehensive review. Applied Biosciences 2024;3(4).
19. Aiga A, Asaumi K, Lee YJ, et al. Expression of neurotrophins and their receptors tropomyosin-related kinases (Trk) under tension-stress during distraction osteogenesis. Acta Med Okayama 2006;60(5):267–77.
20. Nogueira MP, Paley D. Prophylactic and therapeutic peroneal nerve decompression for deformity correction and lengthening. Operat Tech Orthop 2011;21(2):180–3.
21. Compton J, Fragomen A, Rozbruch SR. Skeletal repair in distraction osteogenesis: mechanisms and enhancements. JBJS Rev 2015;3(8):e2.
22. Lumpkin CK Jr, Aronson J, Shen XC, et al. The impact of total enteral nutrition on distraction osteogenesis in a rat model. J Bone Miner Res 1996;11(7):962–9.
23. Hvid I, Horn J, Huhnstock S, et al. The biology of bone lengthening. J Child Orthop 2016;10(6):487–92.
24. Bafor A, Isler A, Sprangel K, et al. Qualitative and quantitative assessment of the regenerate bone formed during intramedullary limb lengthening using a goat (Caprine) Tibia model: a pilot study. Journal of Limb Lengthening & Reconstruction 2024;10(2):78–85.
25. Sun XT, Easwar TR, Stephen M, et al. Comparative study of callus progression in limb lengthening with or without intramedullary nail with reference to the pixel value ratio and the Ru Li's classification. Arch Orthop Trauma Surg 2011;131(10):1333–40.
26. Aronson J, Shen X. Experimental healing of distraction osteogenesis comparing metaphyseal with diaphyseal sites. Clin Orthop Relat Res 1994;301:25–30.
27. Dabis J, Templeton-Ward O, Lacey AE, et al. The history, evolution and basic science of osteotomy techniques. Strategies Trauma Limb Reconstr 2017;12(3):169–80.
28. Eralp L, Kocaoğlu M, Ozkan K, et al. A comparison of two osteotomy techniques for tibial lengthening. Arch Orthop Trauma Surg 2004;124(5):298–300.
29. Lee DH, Ryu KJ, Kim JW, et al. Bone marrow aspirate concentrate and platelet-rich plasma enhanced bone healing in distraction osteogenesis of the tibia. Clin Orthop Relat Res 2014;472(12):3789–97.
30. Sabharwal S. Enhancement of bone formation during distraction osteogenesis: pediatric applications. J Am Acad Orthop Surg 2011;19(2):101–11.
31. Ilizarov GA. The tension-stress effect on the genesis and growth of tissues: part II. The influence of the rate and frequency of distraction. Clin Orthop Relat Res 1989;239:263–85.
32. Morrison SG, Georgiadis AG, Huser AJ, et al. Complications of limb lengthening with motorized intramedullary nails. J Am Acad Orthop Surg 2020;28(18):e803–9.
33. Djasim UM, Mathot BJ, Wolvius EB, et al. Histomorphometric comparison between continuous and discontinuous distraction osteogenesis. J Cranio-Maxillofacial Surg 2009;37(7):398–404.
34. Bright AS, Herzenberg JE, Paley D, et al. Preliminary experience with motorized distraction for tibial lengthening. Strategies Trauma Limb Reconstr 2014;9(2):97–100.
35. Liu Z, Liu Q, Guo H, et al. Overview of physical and pharmacological therapy in enhancing bone regeneration formation during distraction osteogenesis. Front Cell Dev Biol 2022;10:837430.
36. Bafor A, Duncan ME, Iobst CA. Evaluating the utility of the pixel value ratio in the determination of time to full weight-bearing in patients undergoing intramedullary limb lengthening. Strategies Trauma Limb Reconstr 2020;15(2):74–8.
37. Wu C, Huang Y, Huang P, et al. New bone formation accelerates during lower limb lengthening and deformity correction in children with Ollier's disease. J Orthop Traumatol 2023;24(1):39.
38. Bafor A, Iobst C, Samchukov M, et al. Reverse dynamization accelerates regenerate bone formation and remodeling in a goat distraction osteogenesis model. J Bone Joint Surg Am 2023;105(24):1937–46.
39. Fragomen AT, Rozbruch SR. The mechanics of external fixation. HSS J 2007;3(1):13–29.
40. Baruah RK, Patowary S. Accordion maneuver: a bloodless tool in Ilizarov. Journal of Limb Lengthening & Reconstruction 2018;4(1):11–9.
41. Makhdom AM, Cartaleanu AS, Rendon JS, et al. The accordion maneuver: a noninvasive strategy for absent or delayed callus formation in cases of limb lengthening. Adv Orthop 2015;2015:912790.
42. Ren Z, Yang J, Wang Z, et al. Ilizarov method combined with accordion technique for treating long bone defects in the lower limbs: a systematic review. J Orthop Surg Res 2024;19(1):781.
43. Gebauer D, Correll J. Pulsed low-intensity ultrasound: a new salvage procedure for delayed unions and nonunions after leg lengthening in children. J Pediatr Orthop 2005;25(6):750–4.
44. Hankenson KD, Dishowitz M, Gray C, et al. Angiogenesis in bone regeneration. Injury 2011;42(6):556–61.
45. Salem KH, Schmelz A. Low-intensity pulsed ultrasound shortens the treatment time in tibial distraction osteogenesis. Int Orthop 2014;38(7):1477–82.
46. Luna Gonzalez F, Lopez Arévalo R, Meschian CS, et al. Pulsed electromagnetic stimulation of regenerate bone in lengthening procedures. Acta Orthop Belg 2005;71(5):571–6.

47. Eyres KS, Saleh M, Kanis JA. Effect of pulsed electromagnetic fields on bone formation and bone loss during limb lengthening. Bone 1996;18(6):505–9.
48. Narasaki K, Shimizu H, Beppu M, et al. Effect of extracorporeal shock waves on callus formation during bone lengthening. J Orthop Sci 2003;8(4):474–81.
49. Kitoh H, Kitakoji T, Tsuchiya H, et al. Transplantation of culture expanded bone marrow cells and platelet rich plasma in distraction osteogenesis of the long bones. Bone 2007;40(2):522–8.
50. Kiely P, Ward K, Bellemore CM, et al. Bisphosphonate rescue in distraction osteogenesis: a case series. J Pediatr Orthop 2007;27(4):467–71.
51. Aleksyniene R, Thomsen JS, Eckardt H, et al. Parathyroid hormone PTH(1-34) increases the volume, mineral content, and mechanical properties of regenerated mineralizing tissue after distraction osteogenesis in rabbits. Acta Orthop 2009;80(6):716–23.
52. Kudoh A. [Effects of hyperbaric oxygen treatment on healing of maxillary distraction osteogenesis in beagle dogs]. Kokubyo Gakkai Zasshi 2008;75(1):55–64.
53. Atesalp AS, Yurttas Y, Kose O, et al. Effects of hyperbaric oxygen therapy on rabbit skeletal muscle during extremity lengthening. Arch Orthop Trauma Surg 2009;129(1):13–20.

Foot and Ankle

Orthobiologics for Foot and Ankle Tendinopathy

Kristina Quirolgico, MD, FAAPMR, CAQSM[a,b,*],
Garry W.K. Ho, MD, FAMSSM, CAQSM, RMSK[c,d,e,f,g,h], Jessalynn Adam, MD, CAQSM[g,i]

KEYWORDS

- Orthobiologics • Foot • Ankle • Tendinopathy • PRP • Shockwave therapy • Prolotherapy • Regenerative

KEY POINTS

- There is growing evidence-based rationale for orthobiologics in the management of foot and ankle tendinopathies as safe, cost-effective, and minimally invasive therapies.
- Evidence for prolotherapy is limited to treatment of Achilles tendinosis and plantar fasciopathy, but provides rationale for a relatively safe and inexpensive orthobiologic option.
- Platelet-rich plasma and extracorporeal shockwave therapy are treatments for Achilles tendinosis and plantar fasciopathy, but more evidence is needed for use in other foot/ankle tendons.
- Bone marrow aspirate concentrate, microfragmented adipose tissue, amniotic-placental derivatives are potential therapies, but outcomes are limited, and caution should be exercised for use in treatment of foot/ankle tendons.

INTRODUCTION

Foot and ankle tendinopathies are common problems encountered by a variety of health care providers.[1] While most of these conditions respond well to conservative management—activity modification, medications, bracing and orthoses, physical modalities, rehabilitation, and injectable pharmacotherapies—unsatisfactory results often leads to the search for additional treatment options, including surgery. However, for many—including those wishing to avoid surgery—there exists a "treatment gap" between surgery and traditional conservative management. Orthobiologics—a type of "regenerative medicine," defined as the use of biologic therapies in the treatment of musculoskeletal conditions—promises to aid in filling this treatment gap.

From advances in skin grafting, transplant medicine, and tissue engineering, modern regenerative medicine found its roots in the mid-late twentieth century.[2] The term "Orthobiologics" appeared in the 1990s,[3] and over the following decades, began to define the use of regenerative medicine in the treatment of musculoskeletal and neuromuscular conditions. Orthobiologics aim to use molecular biology to steer host cell responses, to re-establish or improve tissue homeostasis and function. In contrast to pharmacotherapy, which uses manufactured, chemical drugs or ligands to provide the central mechanism of therapeutic action, orthobiologics involve the use of biological products—cells, molecules, and biomechanical modalities—to provide the mechanism of therapeutic action.[4] Orthobiologics can come from

[a] Department of Orthopaedic Surgery and Biomedical Engineering, University of Tennessee Health Science Center, Memphis, TN, USA; [b] Campbell Clinic, Germantown, TN, USA; [c] University of Virginia School of Medicine, Charlottesville, VA, USA; [d] Virginia Commonwealth University School of Medicine, Richmond, VA, USA; [e] Georgetown University School of Medicine, Washington, DC, USA; [f] Uniformed Services University of Health Sciences, Bethesda, MD, USA; [g] National Capital Sports Medicine Consortium, Bethesda, MD, USA; [h] OrthoVirginia, Fairfax, VA, USA; [i] OrthoVirginia, Alexandria, VA, USA
* Corresponding author. Campbell Clinic Orthopaedics, 1400 S Germantown Road, Germantown, TN 38138.
E-mail address: kriqui@gmail.com

Orthop Clin N Am 57 (2026) 359–370
https://doi.org/10.1016/j.ocl.2026.06.001

Abbreviations	
AOFAS	American Orthopaedic Foot and Ankle Society
BMAC	bone marrow aspirate concentrate
c-hAM	cryopreserved human amniotic membrane
EFD	energy flux density
ESWT	extracorporeal shockwave therapy
FAOS	Foot and Ankle Outcome Scores
f-ESWT	focused ESWT
FFI	Foot Function Index
GFs	growth factors
IGF-1	insulin-like growth factor–1
IL	interleukin
LP-PRP	leukocyte-poor PRP
LR-PRP	leukocyte-rich PRP
MFAT	microfragmented adipose tissue
MSCs	mesenchymal stromal cells
NO	nitric oxide
NS	normal saline
PPP	platelet-poor plasma
PRP	platelet-rich plasma
PT	physical therapy
RCT	randomized-controlled trial
r-ESWT	radial ESWT
TGF-β	transforming growth factor-beta
VAS	visual analog scales
VISA-A	Victorian Institute of Sport Assessment–Achilles

the patient's own (autologous) or from donor (allogeneic) tissues. These techniques and technologies use a target tissue's local biomolecular resources to overcome the hostile microenvironment responsible for the pathologic state of that tissue. For tendinopathies, orthobiologics seek to turn deterioration and catabolic breakdown into anabolic repair and remodeling.

While orthobiologics may have a role in both acute and chronic tendinopathies, they are primarily used for chronic tendon degeneration and angiofibroblastic disrepair—"tendinosis"—rather than acute inflammation—"tendonitis."[5] This distinction is important because the pathological environments differ between these two disease states, influencing the mechanisms of action of various orthobiologic therapies and, consequently, which therapies should be used and how they should be applied. Additionally, tendinopathies primarily involving different parts and locations of the tendon organ—for example, tendon substance, enthesis, paratenon, or tenosynovium—may also warrant consideration when selecting the optimal treatment approach.

As the technology, techniques, and clinical evidence for orthobiologics continue to develop and advance rapidly, several biologic therapies are available for the treatment of foot and ankle tendinopathies. This article provides a brief overview of the most used orthobiologics.

Prolotherapy

Prolotherapy has been used to treat musculoskeletal conditions for well over a century and is likely the earliest injectable orthobiologic. In the early nineteenth century, general surgeons used organic irritants to treat temporomandibular joint laxity, with multiple other uses reported since the late 1930s.[6] Systematic technique application of prolotherapy was then documented by George S. Hackett[7] in the 1950s. Prolotherapy's original proposed mechanism of action derives from "irritant damage" resulting from injection of the prolotherapy agent (the "proliferant"), initiating the inflammatory cascade by attracting granulocytes and macrophages to remove cellular debris and secrete growth factors (GFs), attracting fibroblasts to the target site.[8] In this way, prolotherapy is aimed at eliciting a local wound-healing response, as fibroblasts produce new collagen, which contracts and remodels into healthier tissue. Several proliferant solutions have been used. Irritants (eg, phenol), chemotactic agents (eg, sodium morrhuate), osmotic agents (eg, hyperosmolar dextrose), and particulates (eg, pumice flour) are 4 types of prolotherapy solutions.[9] While various combinations of proliferants have been used, much of the literature supporting prolotherapy for musculoskeletal applications surrounds the use of hyperosmolar dextrose at concentrations of 10% or higher.[9] Evidence for the efficacy of prolotherapy specifically for the treatment of foot and ankle tendinopathies is limited, but what is currently available does provide rationale for its use.

Achilles tendinopathy

In 2007, Maxwell and colleagues[10] studied prolotherapy in the treatment of Achilles tendinosis in 36 patients with more than 3 months of symptoms. Signs of both midportion and insertional Achilles tendinosis were identified on ultrasound, including neovascularity, increased tendon thickness, effacement of the normally compact-fibrillar sonographic tendon appearance, calcifications, and cortical irregularities. A 25% dextrose solution was injected into the Achilles tendon using ultrasound guidance every 6 weeks until symptoms resolved or no further improvement was shown. The mean number of treatment sessions was 4. Improvements in pain on visual analog scales (VAS) were demonstrated at 6 weeks and 12 months after treatment. Sonographic echogenicity improved in 6 out of 33 tendons, and neovascularity was decreased in 18 out of 33 tendons. No change was found in cortical irregularity or intratendinous calcification.

In 2009, Yelland and colleagues[11] compared eccentric loading exercises and prolotherapy in 40 patients with painful midportion Achilles tendinosis. Fifteen patients entered a 12 week eccentric-loading exercise program. Fourteen patients underwent a prolotherapy injection via hypertonic glucose (20% hyperosmolar dextrose), and 14 patients underwent combined treatment with exercise as well as prolotherapy. Upon analysis of the data, prolotherapy with eccentric loading exercises together demonstrated a more rapid improvement in symptoms than eccentric exercise alone.

In 2010, Ryan and colleagues[12] studied the sonographic appearance of chronic Achilles tendinosis undergoing ultrasound-guided dextrose injections. The study included 86 patients with midportion Achilles tendinosis and 22 patients with insertional tendinosis. A 25% dextrose-lidocaine solution was injected into the tendon via ultrasound guidance. Two years later, the tendon was sonographically evaluated. An appreciable decrease was noted in the size and severity of hypoechoic regions, intratendinous tears, as well as an improvement in neovascularity. This study also reported pain reduction in both groups.

Plantar fasciopathy

In 2020, Mansiz-Kaplan and colleagues[13] published a double-blind randomized-controlled trial (RCT) studying prolotherapy injections for resistant plantar fasciopathy (fasciosis). Patients were randomized to 1 of 2 groups—the prolotherapy group receiving injections of a 15% dextrose solution, or a control group receiving injections of normal saline (NS). Injections were performed twice, 3 weeks apart, with follow-up at 0, 7, and 15 weeks after the interventions, and measuring VAS pain scores during activity and at rest, the Foot Function Index (FFI), and plantar fascia thickness on ultrasonography. Symptom and functional scores, and plantar fascia thickness changes, were significantly greater in the prolotherapy group compared with the control group at 7 and 15 weeks.

In 2026, Vakharia and colleagues[14] also reported an RCT evaluating prolotherapy for plantar fasciopathy. Sixty patients, with symptomatic plantar fasciopathy for at least 6 weeks, were randomized into 2 groups—exercises alone, or exercises and two 15% dextrose injections, 2 weeks apart. VAS pain scores, FFI, and Foot and Ankle Outcome Scores (FAOS) were obtained at 6, 12, and 16 weeks. For the 60 patients completing follow-ups, the prolotherapy group showed significantly better VAS scores at 16 weeks, and better FFI and FAOS scores at both 12 and 16 weeks, compared to the exercise-alone group.

No serious side effects have been found from prolotherapy in the literature. Common temporary side effects include bruising, swelling, pain, and stiffness at the injection site. While more research is needed, prolotherapy is inexpensive relative to other orthobiologics, favoring its use as a cost-effective treatment option for many patients with chronic foot and ankle tendinopathies.

Platelet-rich Plasma

Platelet-rich plasma (PRP) is blood plasma devoid of red blood cells and with a platelet concentration higher than that of whole blood.[15] Platelets modulate inflammation and the healing cascade via the release of cytokines, GFs, and chemokines.[15] Release of bioactive signaling proteins leads to activation of mesenchymal stromal cells (MSCs), monocytes, and fibroblasts, which then promote the removal of degenerative tissue while facilitating healing.[16] PRP is commonly categorized as leukocyte-rich (LR-PRP) or leukocyte-poor (LP-PRP). Tendinopathy has been treated primarily with LR-PRP, as leukocytes help stimulate the repair process, but recent studies found that the ratio of platelets to leukocytes may be more important for healing.[16,17] There are no reported differences between LR-PRP and LP-PRP in mediating nociceptive pain.[17] It has been proposed that considering the leukocyte subpopulation may be important, favoring monocyte-rich, neutrophil-poor PRP for orthobiologic applications.[18]

While there are various methods, PRP is most commonly prepared using a "buffy coat" technique. Venous blood is drawn, followed by centrifugation to separate the whole blood into layers by relative density.[19,20] A major limitation of PRP research is the lack of standardization of PRP formulation across studies, making direct comparisons of study outcomes challenging. In addition, platelet concentration can vary within an individual over time, which can affect the samples obtained and potentially patient outcomes.[16]

Achilles tendinopathy

There is mixed evidence for PRP treatment of Achilles tendinopathy. Most studies focus on midsubstance Achilles tendinopathy, and the majority shows no significant long-term difference between placebo and PRP groups.[21–24] A 2023 meta-analysis by Vithran and colleagues[23] analyzed 8 RCTs where subjects received placebo or PRP injection for Achilles tendinopathy. There was significant improvement in VAS scores in the PRP group compared to the placebo group at 12 weeks, but not at 6 or 24 weeks. While Victorian Institute of Sport Assessment–Achilles (VISA-A) and return-to-sport scores were higher in the PRP group, they were not statistically significant.[23] A 2024 meta-analysis by Ling and colleagues[24] evaluated 6 studies comparing chronic midportion Achilles tendinopathy treated with PRP injection versus placebo, high-volume peritendinous injection, eccentric exercise only, or stromal vascular fraction injections. No significant differences in VISA-A scores between the groups were observed at any time point, and while there was a trend toward reduction in Achilles tendon thickness in the PRP groups, this was not statistically significant.

There are only 2 studies examining the effect of PRP on insertional Achilles tendinopathy, and both compared PRP injection to extracorporeal shockwave therapy (ESWT) rather than placebo.[25,26] These are discussed in the ESWT section of this article.

Anterior and posterior tibial tendinopathy

While there are no RCTs for the use of PRP in anterior or posterior tibial tendinopathy, there is one case series examining anterior tibial tendinopathy. Desomer and colleagues[27] performed a prospective cohort study of 18 patients with anterior tibial tendinopathy. LP-PRP was injected via ultrasound guidance around the tendon insertion, subsequently patients were placed in walking casts for 3 weeks, followed by eccentric strengthening and calf stretching. There were significant improvements in VAS, FFI, and American Orthopaedic Foot and Ankle Society (AOFAS) scores at 6 weeks and 12 weeks compared to baseline.

Peroneal tendinopathy

There is no robust evidence for the use of PRP in peroneal tendinopathy. There was 1 prospective, nonrandomized study by Repetyuk and colleagues[28] of 60 male athletes with peroneal tendinopathy. One group received physical therapy (PT) and ultrasound-guided PRP injection and the other group did PT alone. There was a statistically significant improvement in pain in the PT + PRP group compared to PT alone by 28 days, and return-to-sport was achieved 10 days sooner in the PT + PRP group than in the PT-only group.[28]

Plantar fasciopathy

There are several high-level studies regarding the use of PRP for treatment of plantar fasciopathy. Ye and colleagues[29] performed a meta-analysis of 27 studies, 10 of which were plantar fasciopathy studies comparing PRP to corticosteroid injection. They found similar improvements in VAS pain, AOFAS, and FFI scores in the PRP and corticosteroid groups at 1 and 3 months, but the PRP groups had significantly greater reduction in VAS pain and improvement in functional outcome scores at 6 months. Zuo and colleagues[30] had similar findings in their meta-analysis of 24 plantar fasciopathy studies that compared PRP to corticosteroid injection. The PRP groups had significantly greater improvement in VAS pain scores than the corticosteroid groups at 3 and 6 months, but not 1 or 12 months. The PRP groups also had better AOFAS scores than corticosteroid groups at 3, 6, and 12 months, but no difference between groups at 1 month.[30] There were no differences in plantar fascia thickness between groups at all time points.[30] A 2024 meta-analysis by Herber and colleagues[31] of 21 RCTs compared PRP injection to placebo, corticosteroid injection, prolotherapy, trigger point injections, phonophoresis, and ESWT in treatment of plantar fasciopathy. They found PRP injection resulted in significantly greater improvements in VAS scores compared to corticosteroid injection, ESWT, and placebo.[31] For FFI and plantar fascia thickness, PRP had significantly greater improvement compared to phonophoresis, but not compared to the other treatments.

Summary

Current evidence suggests that PRP injection is a viable treatment option for patients with refractory plantar fasciopathy. There is mixed evidence supporting use in Achilles tendinopathy and further large RCTs are necessary before recommending PRP for use in other foot and ankle tendinopathies.

Platelet-poor Plasma

Platelet-poor plasma (PPP) consists of blood plasma without erythrocytes or leukocytes, has a lower platelet concentration compared to whole blood, and a lower overall GF concentration compared to PRP.[32] PPP has high concentrations of insulin-like growth factor–1 (IGF-1) and hepatocyte growth factor, which may inhibit inflammation and fibrosis, as well as support tissue repair and wound healing.[32] PPP has lower concentrations of transforming growth factor-beta (TGF-β) and myostatin, which was found to decrease proliferation rate but induce myoblast differentiation, which ultimately may better enhance muscle healing.[33]

PPP is obtained through a similar process as PRP. PPP constitutes the least dense layer with a platelet concentration of less than 10,000 platelets/μL and minimal-to-no leukocytes.[19,20]

Clinically, PPP has been used for acute muscle strains given the ability of its constituents to stimulate muscle healing. Currently, there are no RCTs or prospective cohort studies regarding the use of PPP for Achilles or other foot/ankle tendinopathy.

One randomized, double-blind study by Malahias and colleagues[34] compared ultrasound-guided injection of PRP to PPP in patients with chronic plantar fasciopathy. Both groups had a single ultrasound-guided injection of either PRP or PPP. There were statistically significant improvements in pain and functional outcome scores in both groups, and no differences between groups at 3 or 6 months. This outcome suggests that plasma proteins present within both PRP and PPP, not just platelets, may have a role in symptomatic improvement.

More robust studies need to be done, and currently the authors caution the use of PPP in foot and ankle tendinopathy or plantar fasciopathy.

Bone Marrow Aspirate Concentrate

Bone marrow aspirate concentrate (BMAC) is another novel orthobiologic therapy for the treatment of musculoskeletal conditions. BMAC is thought to facilitate tissue repair and healing by promoting cellular proliferation and angiogenesis while also inhibiting proinflammatory cytokines and bacteria.[35] BMAC is derived from bone marrow aspirated from the iliac crest using a Tuohy needle to obtain both cellular and blood products. Density gradient centrifugation is used to concentrate the sample, yielding a mixture of multipotent MSCs, GFs, and PRP, which can promote healing.[36] Actual stem cells contained in BMAC are typically less than 0.01% of the aspirate.[36] While there is great interest in the use of BMAC in both operative and nonoperative settings to improve, augment, or accelerate tissue healing and repair, there is a dearth of literature regarding the use of BMAC for the foot and ankle tendon pathology.

There is a single study investigating the use of BMAC for the nonsurgical management of Achilles tendinopathy. One retrospective chart review by Thueakthong and colleagues[37] for patients with an average of greater than 2 years of symptoms demonstrated improved patient-reported pain scores at all time points from 6 to 48 weeks following injection of BMAC from the iliac crest. They did not report any complications and observed response in both insertional and non-insertional Achilles tendinopathy. This study is limited by small size, retrospective nature, and lack of a control group but demonstrates proof-of-concept for safety and potential efficacy of BMAC as a potential therapy for longstanding recalcitrant Achilles pathology. More research is needed before recommending this therapy. Additionally, there is interest in using BMAC for its potential to augment Achilles tendon repair when performed operatively, however, this extends beyond the scope of this review article.[38]

Similarly, there is one retrospective chart review evaluating the effects of BMAC for chronic plantar fasciopathy.[39] Nineteen patients with an average of 2.5 year history of plantar fasciopathy received an injection of autologous BMAC from the iliac crest at the site of maximal tenderness in the plantar fascia.[39] Following the injection, VAS scores were significantly improved by 6 weeks with statistically diminished VAS score persisting through the final timepoint of 48 weeks.[39] There are notable limitations of this study inherent to a retrospective chart review including small sample size, retrospective nature of the study, lack of a randomization and blinding, lack of control group, and absence of additional functional and objective outcome measures. Additional high-quality studies are needed before recommending BMAC for foot and ankle tendon pathology.

Microfragmented Adipose Tissue

Microfragmented adipose tissue (MFAT) has emerged as an alternative source of autologous MSCs to BMAC for the treatment of musculoskeletal conditions. MFAT can be obtained in the clinical setting by inserting a 17 g trocar into the subcutaneous abdominal or flank adipose tissue layers and injecting a tumescent solution, after which a separate trocar is inserted and passed back and forth through the tissue to break down the adipose, and during this step, negative pressure is applied to obtain a lipoaspirate sample.[40] Typically, this process is repeated until about 40 mL of total lipoaspirate is collected, which is then rinsed using an NS solution, and filtered to obtain a final MFAT product.[40] Some processing protocols may include further mechanical resizing of the adipose tissues, but this varies across MFAT systems. The final MFAT product can then be injected at the site of pathology. MFAT is particularly promising for tendon pathology given its proposed anti-inflammatory and proliferative effects.[41] MFAT is thought to prevent tissue fibrosis and catabolism by enhancing the production of GFs, such as vascular endothelial growth factor (VEGF), interleukin-1 receptor antagonist (IL-1Ra), interleukin-6 while simultaneously blocking the inflammatory effects of interleukin-1 beta (IL-1β) on tendons.[41] Current US federal regulatory guidelines mandate minimal manipulation of this adipose, forbidding further biological processing of the specimen outside of special licensing requirements or as part of an investigational trial.

There is very little research on the use of MFAT for foot and ankle pathology. Much of the research on MFAT was pioneered by the late Gerard Malanga, MD, and the New Jersey Regenerative Institute. His group published a single case report on the use of MFAT injection for chronic intrasubstance Achilles tendon defects.[42] The patient had clinical concerns of pain and weakness for greater than 1 year and was treated with MFAT via sonographically guided injection.[42] Four weeks posttreatment, the patient had returned to his regular activities and continued to be pain-free at 6 months of follow-up.[42]

Extracorporeal Shockwave Therapy

ESWT is a noninvasive treatment of various musculoskeletal issues. The proposed mechanism of action is through microcavitation resulting from acoustic waves passing through tissues, which may stimulate interstitial and extracellular healing responses (**Table 1**).[43–45] ESWT is also thought to have a separate analgesic effect, though the exact mechanism is not fully understood (see **Table 1**).[43,44] ESWT is noninvasive and typically well tolerated. The most commonly reported side effects are temporary local pain, skin bruising, and erythema.[43,44,46] ESWT is primarily described in literature as 2 types, focused (f-ESWT) and radial (r-ESWT) shockwave therapy. f-ESWT is generated by electrohydraulic, electromagnetic, and piezoelectric devices.[44,45] r-ESWT is produced via pneumatic compression devices.[44,45] Recently, r-ESWT have been referred to as radial pressure waves as they are generated via mechanotransduction at lower speed and peak pressure compared to f-ESWT.[44,45] They have maximum effect superficially, then attenuate as they travel deeper into the tissue.[45] There are various parameters that can be adjusted depending on the patient and condition being treated (**Table 2**).[44,45] Focused shockwaves converge with a treatment-zone depth up to 5 to 6 cm, depending on the manufacturer.[44,45] An advantage of ESWT is the ability to treat multiple areas in a single session. For example, treatment can be performed on the entire muscle–tendon–bone unit (eg, for Achilles tendinopathy, targeting the gastrocnemius muscles and Achilles tendon at the midportion and/or insertion).[45] Studies have shown that clinical focusing—treating areas with the most pain—has been just as effective as image-guidance for most conditions, though the combination can be helpful for targeting deeper tissues.[44,45] Use of anesthetic should be avoided as this decreases efficacy.[44,45] Variability in ESWT settings and protocols has resulted in considerable heterogeneity across published clinical outcomes.

Achilles tendinopathy

There is mixed evidence regarding the use of ESWT for Achilles tendinopathy. A meta-analysis by Fan and colleagues[47] evaluated 8 studies including subjects with midportion and insertional Achilles tendinopathy, comparing ESWT to placebo or eccentric strengthening exercises. ESWT groups noted greater improvement in pain and functional outcome scores (VISA-A, AOFAS, Roles and Maudsley) up to 12 months compared to other groups. Ni and colleagues[48] performed a meta-analysis of 8 studies comparing ESWT to placebo for treating chronic Achilles tendinopathy. There was heterogeneity across studies with 4 using r-ESWT, 3 using f-ESWT, 3 to 4 sessions over 4 to 6 weeks, 1500 to 4500 pulses per session, and low to high energy intensity. There was significant pain reduction in the ESWT group at 1 and 3 months compared to placebo if their symptoms were less than 12 months duration.[48] There were no significant differences in functional outcomes between groups, nor were there significant differences between tendinopathy classification or ESWT type.[48] In 2023, Bai and colleagues[25] compared PRP injection to ESWT in the treatment of insertional Achilles tendinopathy. They found that VAS and VISA-A scores significantly improved in both groups by 1, 3, and 6 months, with the PRP

Table 1
Proposed mechanisms of action of extracorporeal shockwave therapy

Mechanism	Biological Effect	Clinical Relevance
Neovascularization/ Angiogenesis	Upregulation of vascular endothelial growth factor (VEGF), endothelial nitric oxide synthase (eNOS), and proliferating cell nuclear antigen (PCNA)	Improves local blood supply and tissue healing
Stem/Progenitor cell activation	Recruitment and differentiation of mesenchymal stem cells	Enhances healing potential of damaged tissue
Growth factor release	Increased TGF-β, IGF-1, platelet-derived growth factor (PDGF), and bone morphogenetic proteins (BMPs)	Promotes matrix synthesis and repair
Anti-inflammatory effects	Downregulation of IL-1β, tumor necrosis factor-alpha, and cyclooxygenase-2 (COX-2)	Reduces chronic inflammatory signaling
Nitric oxide (NO) production	Increased NO synthase activity	Improves microcirculation and modulates inflammation
Pain modulation (neurogenic)	Reduced substance P, calcitonin gene-related peptide (CGRP); altered nociceptor activity	Analgesic effect independent of structural healing
Hyperstimulation analgesia	Overstimulation of pain receptors	Short-term pain relief
Cavitation/Microtrauma	Controlled microinjury to tissue	Restarts stalled healing cascade in chronic tendinopathy
Matrix remodeling	Increased collagen type I synthesis, tenocyte proliferation	Improves tendon structure and mechanical strength

Table 2
Extracorporeal shockwave therapy parameters

Parameter	Typical Range/Description	Notes/Clinical Relevance
ESWT type	Focused (f-ESWT) or radial (r-ESWT)	Focused can target deeper tissues; radial is more superficial
Energy flux density (EFD)	0.05–0.55 mJ/mm^2	Low (<0.1), medium (0.1–0.28), and high (>0.28)
Pressure (r-ESWT)	0–5.0 bar	Reported instead of EFD for r-ESWT, however true EFD conversion cannot be directly standardized across devices; in general low (up to ~2.0 bar), medium (~2.0–4.5 bar)
# Shocks per session	1500–4000 pulses	Most studies use ~2000–3000
Frequency	3–21 Hz	Higher frequencies shorten treatment time
Number of Sessions	1–5	Commonly 3 sessions
Interval between sessions	5–14 d	Weekly is most typical
Localization method	Ultrasound-guided or clinical focusing	U/S improves precision for deep pathology
Anesthesia	None	Avoiding anesthesia is recommended to improve biological effect
Coupling medium	Ultrasound gel	Required for energy transmission

group having better scores at 6 months compared to the ESWT group. Erroi and colleagues[26] performed a retrospective comparison between PRP injection and focused ESWT for insertional Achilles tendinopathy and found that both groups improved at 2, 4, and 6 months. PRP injections were performed under ultrasound guidance once a week for 2 weeks. ESWT was administered over 3 weeks at 0.17 to 0.25 mJ/mm^2, 2400 pulses, titrated up to patient tolerance.[26] The ESWT group had a higher VISA-A score at 4 months; otherwise, there were no statistically significant differences between groups at other time points.[26]

Anterior and posterior tibial tendinopathy, peroneal tendinopathy

There are currently no high-level studies regarding the use of ESWT in anterior or posterior tibial tendinopathy or peroneal tendinopathy. There is one small case series by Robinson and colleagues[49] where 10 subjects with posterior tibial tendinopathy were treated with at least 3 weekly sessions of r-ESWT combined with foot core exercises. They had significant improvement in functional outcome scores by 4 months.

Plantar fasciopathy

Most robust evidence for ESWT is in plantar fasciopathy; however, there is significant variability in published protocols.

A meta-analysis of 16 RCTs performed by Cortés-Pérez and colleagues[46] in 2024 compared ESWT to corticosteroid injection. There was statistically greater improvement in pain and foot function in the ESWT groups at 3 and 6 months, and plantar fascia thickness was significantly decreased in the ESWT group at 3 months compared to the corticosteroid group. Daher and colleagues[50] did a meta-analysis of 6 RCTs comparing PRP injection to ESWT in plantar fasciopathy. Groups receiving PRP injection had statistically greater reduction in pain and plantar fascia thickness compared to ESWT. Tung and colleagues[51] performed a meta-analysis in 2025 of 15 studies comparing ESWT to placebo, PT, custom orthotics, corticosteroid injection, prolotherapy, and PRP injection. There was a statistically significant improvement in VAS scores in the ESWT group compared to placebo, less improvement compared to PRP, and no differences compared to other treatments. ESWT had significantly greater improvements in FFI compared to corticosteroid injection, less improvement compared to PRP and custom orthotics, and no differences compared to other treatments.[51] There were no differences between groups regarding plantar fascia thickness change.[51]

There are parameters when performing ESWT that can be adjusted to optimize patient experience and outcomes. One variable is energy intensity. Zhao and colleagues[52] evaluated whether differing energy intensity levels resulted in better outcomes in participants with heel pain. They did a meta-analysis of 22 RCTs and found that medium-intensity and high-intensity ESWT resulted in greater reduction in pain compared to placebo, and there were no significant differences between the 2 energy intensities. There were no statistically significant differences between low-intensity ESWT and placebo in pain reduction.[52] In terms of functional outcomes, medium-intensity ESWT was superior to placebo and low-intensity ESWT, but there was no difference compared to high-intensity ESWT.[52]

Summary

Based on the current evidence, ESWT may reduce pain in those with Achilles tendinopathy symptoms less than 12 months. ESWT may improve pain and function in insertional Achilles tendinopathy and plantar fasciopathy at midterm, though PRP has better outcomes. When performing ESWT for plantar fasciopathy and Achilles tendinopathy, it is recommended to use medium-intensity energy levels. There is not enough evidence to support the use of ESWT for other foot/ankle tendinopathies. While there is currently no evidence of significant differences in outcomes between f-ESWT and r-ESWT, forthcoming studies are evaluating whether combination treatment of f-ESWT and r-ESWT results in superior outcomes compared to either alone.

Amniotic Membrane/Placental Derivatives

Amniotic membrane and placental-derived products are used across multiple specialties for their ability to promote wound healing. They have piqued interest for use in the treatment of musculoskeletal pathologies. They are a potential source of pluripotent cells, collagen matrix proteins, immunomodulators, and anti-inflammatory cytokines.[53] While there are numerous articles detailing the basic science and nonorthopedic applications of these products, there are significantly fewer human studies specific to sports medicine.[53] One small prospective, double-blind single-center RCT of 23 patients was performed in 2014 evaluating the use of cryopreserved human amniotic membrane (c-hAM) for refractory plantar fasciopathy.[54] The control group received a corticosteroid injection and the treatment group received c-hAM. Patients were followed for 18 weeks and the Foot Health Status Questionnaire and VAS were recorded as primary and secondary outcomes.[54] The study found similar outcomes between the treatment and control groups providing a rationale for c-hAM as a potential alternative to corticosteroid injection for plantar fasciopathy.[54] A larger prospective, single-center RCT of 45 patients was performed by Zelen and colleagues.[55] The treatment groups received an injection of 2 mL of 0.5% marcaine followed by an injection of 0.5 or 1.25 mL of dehydrated human amniotic/chorionic membrane (mDHACM), while the control group received the 2 mL of marcaine followed by 1.25 mL of NS. They found improvements in AOFAS Hindfoot scores as early as 1 week after treatment with both mDHACM groups.[55] Another human study of 55 patients with recalcitrant plantar fasciosis and Achilles tendinosis noted improvement following treatment with an allograft of c-hAM and amniotic fluid.[56] However, the study is confounded by the concurrent use of radial shockwave therapy in the treatment protocol.

While there are very few studies investigating the application of placental allografts for foot and ankle pathologies, the limited human data suggest this as an area of additional research worth following for potential orthopedic applications in foot and ankle pathologies. A major criticism of placental products and the limited body of research on placental allografts in orthopedic medicine is the heterogeneity of the placental cell types, variable preparations of products, and lack of consistent treatment regimens across studies.[57] Additionally, commercially available preparations of these products do not contain live cells, and it is important to include this fact when counseling patients interested in pursuing this orthobiologic option.

SUMMARY

Foot and ankle tendinopathies continue to present challenges for patients and health care providers alike, particularly in those with unsatisfactory responses to conservative measures and traditional treatments alone, and those who wish to avoid surgery. While the supporting evidence base is in need of continued development and study, orthobiologics provide a rational and promising option to fill this treatment gap. Prolotherapy, PRP, PPP, BMAC, MFAT, ESWT, and amniotic-placental derivatives remain novel options with potential to improve patient outcomes. It is expected that technical and technological development in orthobiologics will continue at an increasingly rapid pace. However, the regulatory environment in which the clinician practices must be considered in order to employ these therapies in a safe and compliant manner. While the specifics of governmental rules and policies are beyond the scope of this article, the reader is encouraged to exercise sound judgment and best practices in the use of orthobiologics.

CLINICS CARE POINTS

- It is recommended for patients to do PT concurrently while being treated with orthobiologics to improve outcomes.
- While multiple options for prolotherapy solutions are available, hyperosmolar 10% to 25% dextrose is the most well studied and easiest-to-use proliferant.
- Local anesthetic should be avoided when performing ESWT as this can decrease clinical effectiveness.
- BMAC and MFAT are emerging orthobiologic therapies. They must be used with caution to ensure that they are processed with minimal manipulation and for autologous use to comply with Food and Drug Administration regulations.

DECLARATION OF ARTIFICIAL INTELLIGENCE AND ARTIFICIAL INTELLIGENCE-ASSISTED TECHNOLOGIES IN THE WRITING PROCESS

During the preparation of this article, the authors used FigureLabs in order to develop 1 or more illustrative figures. After using this tool/service, the authors reviewed and edited the content as needed and take full responsibility for the content of the publication.

DISCLOSURE

The authors have nothing to disclose.

REFERENCES

1. Jarvinen M. Epidemiology of tendon injuries in sports. Clin Sports Med 1992;11:493–504.
2. Sampogna G, Guraya SY, Forgione A. Regenerative medicine: historical roots and potential strategies in modern medicine. J Microsc Ultrastruct 2015;3(3):101–7.

3. Dhillon MS, Patel S. Why OrthoBiologics? J Clin Orthop Trauma 2022;28:101850.
4. Andia I, Maffulli N. Muscle and tendon injuries: the role of biological interventions to promote and assist healing and recovery. Arthroscopy 2015; 31(5):999–1015.
5. Kraushaar B, Nirschl RP. Current concepts review: tendinosis of the elbow (tennis elbow). Clinical features and findings of histological, immunochemical, and electron microscopy studies. J Bone Joint Surg Am 1999;81:259–78.
6. Schultz L. A treatment for subluxation of the temporomandibular joint. J Am Med Assoc 1937; 109(13):1032–5.
7. Hackett GS, Hemwall GA, Montgomery GA. Ligament and tendon relaxation treated by prolotherapy. Oak Park (IL): Hemwall; 1993. Gustav A.
8. Sharma P, Maffulli N. Biology of tendon injury: healing, modeling and remodeling. J Musculoskelet Neuronal Interact 2006;6(2):181–90.
9. Banks A. A rationale for prolotherapy. J. Orthop. Med 1991;13(3):54–9.
10. Maxwell NJ, Ryan MB, Taunton JE, et al. Sonographically guided intratendinous injection of hyperosmolar dextrose to treat chronic tendinosis of the achilles tendon: a pilot study. Am J Roentgenol 2007;189(4):215–20.
11. Yelland MJ, Sweeting KR, Lyftogt JA, et al. Prolotherapy injections and eccentric loading exercises for painful achilles tendinosis: a randomised trial. Br J Sports Med 2010;45(5):421–8.
12. Ryan M, Wong A, Taunton J. Favorable outcomes after sonographically guided intratendinous injection of hyperosmolar dextrose for chronic insertional and midportion achilles tendinosis. Am J Roentgenol 2010;194(4):1047–53.
13. Mansiz-Kaplan B, Nacir B, Pervane-Vural S, et al. Effect of dextrose prolotherapy on pain intensity, disability, and plantar fascia thickness in unilateral plantar fasciitis: a randomized, controlled, double-blind study. Am J Phys Med Rehabil 2020;99(4): 318–24.
14. Vakharia K, Arya RK, Mohanta S. Effectiveness of dextrose prolotherapy in addition to plantar fascia stretches to plantar fascia stretches alone in the treatment of chronic plantar fasciitis: a randomized-controlled trial. J Arthrosc Surg Sports Med 2026;7:86–91.
15. Finnoff JT, Awan TM, Borg-Stein J, et al. American medical society for sports medicine position statement: principles for the responsible use of regenerative medicine in sports medicine. Clin J Sport Med 2021;31(6):530–41.
16. Foster TE, Puskas BL, Mandelbaum BR, et al. Platelet-rich plasma: from basic science to clinical applications. Am J Sports Med 2009;37(11): 2259–72.
17. Jayaram P, Mitchell PJT, Shybut TB, et al. Leukocyte-rich platelet-rich plasma is predominantly anti-inflammatory compared with leukocyte-poor platelet-rich plasma in patients with mild-moderate knee osteoarthritis: a prospective, descriptive laboratory study. Am J Sports Med 2023;51(8):2133–40.
18. Lana JF, Huber SC, Purita J, et al. Leukocyte-rich PRP versus leukocyte-poor PRP - the role of monocyte/macrophage function in the healing Cascade. J Clin Orthop Trauma 2019;10(Suppl 1):S7–12.
19. Le ADK, Enweze L, DeBaun MR, et al. Platelet-rich plasma. Clin Sports Med 2019;38(1):17–44.
20. Rossi LA, Murray IR, Chu CR, et al. Classification systems for platelet-rich plasma. Bone Joint J 2019;101-B(8):891–6.
21. Bagheri K, Krez A, Anastasio AT, et al. The use of platelet-rich plasma in pathologies of the foot and ankle: a comprehensive review of the recent literature. Foot Ankle Surg 2023;29(8):551–9.
22. Johnson LG, Buck EH, Anastasio AT, et al. Efficacy of platelet-rich plasma in soft tissue foot and ankle pathology. JBJS Rev 2022;10(10) [Erratum in: JBJS Rev. 2022 Nov 2;10(11)].
23. Arthur Vithran DT, Xie W, Opoku M, et al. The efficacy of platelet-rich plasma injection therapy in the treatment of patients with achilles tendinopathy: a systematic review and meta-analysis. J Clin Med 2023;12(3):995.
24. Ling SK-K, Mak CT-K, Lo JP-Y, et al. Effect of platelet-rich plasma injection on the treatment of achilles tendinopathy: a systematic review and meta-analysis. Orthop J Sports Med 2024;12(11): 23259671241296508.
25. Bai WB, Liang XJ, Zhao HM, et al. [Comparison of efficacy of platelet-rich plasma and extracorporeal shock wave for the treatment of chronic insertional achilles tendinopathy]. Zhong Guo Gu Shang 2023; 36(4):351–6.
26. Erroi D, Sigona M, Suarez T, et al. Conservative treatment for insertional achilles tendinopathy: platelet-rich plasma and focused shock waves. A retrospective study. Muscles Ligaments Tendons J 2017;7(1):98–106.
27. Desomer L, van Beek N, Van Riet A, et al. Outcomes of platelet-rich plasma infiltration and weightbearing cast immobilization in distal tibialis anterior tendinopathy: a prospective cohort study. Foot Ankle Int 2024;45(2):158–65.
28. Repetyuk A, Achkasov E, Sereda A. Efficacy of platelet-rich plasma in the rehabilitation of athletes with peroneal tendinopathy: a prospective non-randomized study of 60 patients. Bulletin of Rehabilitation Medicine 2022;21:116–21.
29. Ye Z, Yuan Y, Kuang G, et al. Platelet-rich plasma and corticosteroid injection for tendinopathy: a systematic review and meta-analysis. BMC Musculoskelet Disord 2025;26(1):339.

30. Zuo A, Gao C, Jia Q, et al. Platelet-rich plasma versus corticosteroids in the treatment of plantar fasciitis: a systematic review and meta-analysis. Am J Phys Med Rehabil 2025;104(7):613–21.
31. Herber A, Covarrubias O, Daher M, et al. Platelet rich plasma therapy versus other modalities for treatment of plantar fasciitis: a systematic review and meta-analysis. Foot Ankle Surg 2024;30(4): 285–93.
32. Fernandes GCAM, Rodeo SA. Platelet-poor plasma for muscle injuries: a review of mechanisms and clinical perspectives. Orthop J Sports Med 2025;13-(11):23259671251356628.
33. Miroshnychenko O, Chang WT, Dragoo JL. The use of platelet-rich and platelet-poor plasma to enhance differentiation of skeletal myoblasts: implications for the use of autologous blood products for muscle regeneration. Am J Sports Med 2017; 45(4):945–53.
34. Malahias MA, Mavrogenis AF, Nikolaou VS, et al. Similar effect of ultrasound-guided platelet-rich plasma versus platelet-poor plasma injections for chronic plantar fasciitis. Foot 2019;38:30–3.
35. Blanton CM, Clougherty CO. The role of bone marrow aspirate in osseous and soft tissue pathology. Clin Podiatr Med Surg 2021;38(1):1–16.
36. Shapiro E, Grande D, Drakos M. Biologics in achilles tendon healing and repair: a review. Curr Rev Musculoskelet Med 2015;8(1):9–17.
37. Thueakthong W, de Cesar Netto C, Garnjanagoonchorn A, et al. Outcomes of iliac crest bone marrow aspirate injection for the treatment of recalcitrant achilles tendinopathy. Int Orthop 2021;45(9):2423–8.
38. Imam MA, Holton J, Horriat S, et al. A systematic review of the concept and clinical applications of bone marrow aspirate concentrate in tendon pathology. SICOT J 2017;3:58.
39. de Cesar Netto C, Day J, Auster H, et al. Outcomes of iliac crest bone marrow aspirate injection in the treatment of recalcitrant plantar fasciitis. Int Orthop 2026;50(2):463–7.
40. McGee C, Baria MR, Gatewood C, et al. Lipoaspiration and processing to create microfragmented adipose tissue. Video J Sports Med 2022;2(3): 26350254221076855.
41. Viganò M, Lugano G, Perucca Orfei C, et al. Autologous microfragmented adipose tissue reduces the catabolic and fibrosis response in an in vitro model of tendon cell inflammation. Stem Cells Int 2019;2019:5620286.
42. Iuso AM, Pacik D, Martin J, et al. Adipose cellular injection in the treatment of an intrasubstance achilles tendon defect: a case report. Regen Med 2022;17(11):835–43.
43. Rhim HC, Singh M, Maffulli N, et al. Recommendations for use of extracorporeal shockwave therapy in sports medicine: an international modified Delphi study. Br J Sports Med 2025;59(18):1287–301.
44. Schroeder AN, Tenforde AS, Jelsing EJ. Extracorporeal shockwave therapy in the management of sports medicine injuries. Curr Sports Med Rep 2021;20(6):298–305.
45. Tenforde AS, Borgstrom HE, DeLuca S, et al. Best practices for extracorporeal shockwave therapy in musculoskeletal medicine: clinical application and training consideration. PMR 2022;14(5):611–9.
46. Cortés-Pérez I, Moreno-Montilla L, Ibáñez-Vera AJ, et al. Efficacy of extracorporeal shockwave therapy, compared to corticosteroid injections, on pain, plantar fascia thickness and foot function in patients with plantar fasciitis: a systematic review and meta-analysis. Clin Rehabil 2024;38(8): 1023–43.
47. Fan Y, Feng Z, Cao J, et al. Efficacy of extracorporeal shock wave therapy for achilles tendinopathy: a meta-analysis. Orthop J Sports Med 2020;8(2): 2325967120903430.
48. Ni T, Zhao Y, Pang L, et al. Extracorporeal shockwave therapy versus sham extracorporeal shockwave therapy for chronic achilles tendinopathy: a meta-analysis of randomized-controlled trials. PeerJ 2026;14:e20506.
49. Robinson D, Mitchkash M, Wasserman L, et al. Nonsurgical approach in management of tibialis posterior tendinopathy with combined radial shockwave and foot core exercises: a case series. J Foot Ankle Surg 2020;59(5):1058–61.
50. Daher M, Covarrubias O, Herber A, et al. Platelet-rich plasma vs extracorporeal shock wave therapy in the treatment of plantar fasciitis at 3-6 months: a systematic review and meta-analysis of randomized-controlled trials. Foot Ankle Int 2024; 45(7):796–803.
51. Tung WS, Daher M, Covarrubias O, et al. Extracorporeal shock wave therapy shows comparative results with other modalities for the management of plantar fasciitis: a systematic review and meta-analysis. Foot Ankle Surg 2025;31(4):283–90.
52. Zhao P, He Y, Li M, et al. Comparative efficacy and acceptability of different intensity levels of extracorporeal shock wave therapy in adults with plantar heel pain: a systematic review and network meta-analysis. Pharm Manag PM R 2025;17(12): 1481–93.
53. Riboh JC, Saltzman BM, Yanke AB, et al. Human amniotic membrane–derived products in sports medicine: basic science, early results, and potential clinical applications: basic science, early results, and potential clinical applications. Am J Sports Med 2015;44(9):2425–34.
54. Hanselman AE, Tidwell JE, Santrock RD. Cryopreserved human amniotic membrane injection for plantar fasciitis: a randomized, controlled,

double-blind pilot study. Foot Ankle Int 2015; 36(2):151–8. Epub 2014 Sep 23.
55. Zelen CM, Poka A, Andrews J. Prospective, randomized, blinded, comparative study of injectable micronized dehydrated amniotic/chorionic membrane allograft for plantar fasciitis–a feasibility study. Foot Ankle Int 2013;34(10):1332–9. Epub 2013 Aug 14.
56. Werber B. Amniotic tissues for the treatment of chronic plantar fasciosis and achilles tendinosis. J Sports Med 2015;2015(1):219896.
57. McIntyre JA, Jones IA, Danilkovich A, et al. The placenta: applications in orthopaedic sports medicine. Am J Sports Med 2018;46(1):234–47. Epub 2017 Apr 4.

United States Postal Service

Statement of Ownership, Management and Circulation
(All Periodicals Publications Except Requester Publications)

1. Publication Title	2. Publication Number	3. Filing Date
ORTHOPEDIC CLINICS OF NORTH AMERICA	9 5 0 - 9 2 0	08/24/2026
4. Issue Frequency	**5. Number of Issues Published Annually**	**6. Annual Subscription Price**
JAN, APR, JUL, OCT	4	$376.00

7. Complete Mailing Address of Known Office of Publication (Not printer) (Street, city, county, state, and ZIP+4)

Addr 1: Elsevier INC
Addr 2: 230 Park Ave Ste 800
City, State ZIP: New York NY 10169

Contact Person: Mohana Priya Damodharan
Telephone: 91-44-4299-4077

8. Complete Mailing Address of Headquarters or General Business Office of Publisher (Not Printer)

Addr 1: Elsevier INC
Addr 2: 230 Park Ave Ste 800
City, State ZIP: New York NY 10169

9. Full Names and Complete Mailing Addresses of Publisher, Editor and Managing Editor (do not leave blank)

Publisher (Name and complete mailing address)
Name: Dolores Meloni, ELSEVIER INC.
Addr 1: 1600 JOHN F KENNEDY BLVD. SUITE 1600
Addr 2:
City, State ZIP: PHILADELPHIA, PA 19103-2899

Editor (Name and complete mailing address)
Name: ASHLIE JACKMAN, ELSEVIER INC.
Addr 1: 1ST FLOOR, NIELSEN HOUSE, JOHN SMITH DRIVE
Addr 2:
City, State ZIP: OXFORD, OX4 2WB, UK

Managing Editor (Name and complete mailing address)
Name: PATRICK MANLEY, ELSEVIER INC.
Addr 1: 1600 JOHN F KENNEDY BLVD. SUITE 1600
Addr 2:
City, State ZIP: PHILADELPHIA, PA 19103-2899

10. Owner (Do not leave blank. If the publication is owned by a corporation, give the name and address of the corporation immediately followed by the names and addresses of all stockholders owning or holding 1 Percent or more of the total amount of stock. If not owned by a corporation, give the names and addresses of all the individual owners. If owned by a partnership or other unincorporated firm, give it's name and address as well as those of each individual owner. If the publication is published by a nonprofit organization, give it's name and address.)

Full Name	Complete Mailing Address
WHOLLY OWNED SUBSIDIARY OF REED/ELSEVIER,	1600 JOHN F KENNEDY BLVD. SUITE 1600
US HOLDINGS	PHILADELPHIA, PA 19103-2899

11. Known Bondholders, Mortgagees and Other Security Holders Owning or Holding 1 Percent or more of Total Amount of Bonds, Mortgages, or Other Securities. If none, check box → ☐ None

Full Name	Complete Mailing Address
NA	

12. Tax Status (For completion by nonprofit organizations authorized to mail at nonprofit rates) (Check one)
The purpose, function, and nonprofit status of this organization and the exempt status for federal income tax purposes:
[X] Has Not changed During Preceding 12 Months
[ ] Has Changed During Preceding 12 Months (Publisher must submit explanation of change with this statement below)

PS Form 3526, July 2014

13. Publication Title	14. Issue Date for Circulation Data Below	
ORTHOPEDIC CLINICS OF NORTH AMERICA	October 2026	
15. Extent and Nature of Circulation	**Average No. Copies Each Issue During Preceding 12 Months**	**No. Copies of Single Issue Published Nearest to filing Date**
a. Total Number of Copies (Net press run)	98	92
b. Paid and/or Requested Circulation (1) Mailed Outside-County Paid Subscriptions Stated on PS Form 3541 (Include paid distribution above nominal rate, advertiser's proof copies, and exchange copies)	48	45
(2) Mailed In-County Paid Subscriptions Stated on PS Form 3541 (Include paid distribution above nominal rate, advertiser's proof copies, and exchange copies)	0	0
(3) Paid Distribution Outside the Mails Including Sales Through Dealers and Carriers, Street Vendors, Counter Sales ,and Other Paid Distribution Ouside USPS	41	37
(4) Paid Distribution by Other Classes of Mail Through the USPS (e.g. First-Class Mail)	5	6
c. Total Paid Distribution [Sum of 15b. (1), (2), (3), and (4)] ▶	94	88
d. Free or Nominal Rate Distribution (By Mail and Outside the Mail) (1) Free or Nominal Rate Outside-County Copies Included on PS Form 3541	3	3
(2) Free or Nominal In-County Copies Included on PS Form 3541	0	0
(3) Free or Nominal Rate Copies Mailed at Other Classes Through the USPS (e.g. First-Class Mail)	0	0
(4) Free or Nominal Rate Distribution Outside the Mail (Carriers or other means)	1	1
e. Total Free or Nominal Rate Distribution (Sum of 15d. (1), (2), (3) and (4)) ▶	4	4
f. Total Distribution (Sum of 15c. and 15e.) ▶	98	92
g. Copies not Distributed (See Instructions to Publishers #4 (page #3))	0	0
h. Total (Sum of 15f. and g.) ▶	98	92
i. Percent Paid (15c. Divided by 15f. Times 100) ▶	95.92%	95.65%

* if you are claiming electronic copies, go to line 16 on page 3. If you are not claiming electronic copies, skip to line 17 on page 3.

16. Electronic copy Circulation		
If present, check box →		☐
a. Paid Electronic Copies		
b. Total Paid Print Copies (Line 15c) + Paid Electronic Copies (Line 16a) ▶	94	88
c. Total Print Distribution (Line 15F) + Paid Electronic Copies (Line 16a) ▶	98	92
d. Percentage Paid (Both Print & Electronic Copies (16b divided bt 16c x 100) ▶	95.92%	95.65%

[X] I certify that 50% of all my distribution copies (electronic and Print) are paid above a nominal price

17. Publication of Statement of Ownership
[X] Publication required. Will be printed in the **October 2026** issue of this publication. [ ] Publication not required

18. Signature and Title of Editor, Publisher, Business Manager, or Owner

	Title	Date
Mohana Priya Damodharan	Distribution Controller	8/24/2026

I certify that all information furnished on this form is true and complete. I understand that anyone who furnishes false or misleading information on this form or who omits material or information requested on the form may be subject to criminal sanctions (including fines and imprisonment) and/or civil sanctions (including civil penalties)

PS Form 3526, July 2014

9780443430985